Pain Neurosurgery

NEUROSURGERY BY EXAMPLE

Key Cases and Fundamental Principles

Series edited by: Nathan R. Selden, MD, PhD, FACS, FAAP

Volume 1: Peripheral Nerve Neurosurgery, Wilson & Yang
Volume 2: Surgical Neuro-Oncology, Lonser & Elder
Volume 3: Spinal Neurosurgery, Harrop & Maulucci
Volume 4: Pediatric Neurosurgery, Selden & Baird
Volume 5: Pain Neurosurgery, Sagher, Levin, & Pilitsis

Pain Neurosurgery

Edited by

Oren Sagher, Emily Lehmann Levin, and Julie G. Pilitsis

OXFORD
UNIVERSITY PRESS

OXFORD
UNIVERSITY PRESS

Oxford University Press is a department of the University of Oxford. It furthers the University's objective of excellence in research, scholarship, and education by publishing worldwide. Oxford is a registered trade mark of Oxford University Press in the UK and certain other countries.

Published in the United States of America by Oxford University Press
198 Madison Avenue, New York, NY 10016, United States of America.

CIP data is on file at the Library of Congress
ISBN 978–0–19–088767–4

Contents

Series Editor's Preface

Dear Reader,

I am delighted to introduce this volume of *Neurosurgery by Example: Key Cases and Fundamental Principles.* Neurosurgical training and practice are based on managing a wide range of complex clinical cases with expert knowledge, sound judgment, and skilled technical execution. Our goal in this series is to present exemplary cases in the manner they are actually encountered in the neurosurgical clinic, hospital emergency department, and operating room.

For this volume, Drs. Oren Sagher, Emily Lehmann Levin, and Julie G. Pilitsis invited a broad range of expert contributors to share their extensive wisdom and experience in all major areas of pain neurosurgery. Each chapter contains a classic presentation of an important clinical entity, guiding readers through the assessment and planning, decision making, surgical procedure, after care, and complication management. "Pivot points" illuminate the changes required to manage patients in alternate or atypical situations.

Each chapter also presents lists of pearls for the accurate diagnosis, successful treatment, and effective complication management of each clinical problem. These three focus areas will be especially helpful to neurosurgeons preparing to sit for the American Board of Neurological Surgery oral examination, which bases scoring on these three topics.

Finally, each chapter contains focused reviews of medical evidence and expected outcomes, helpful for counseling patients and setting accurate expectations. Rather than exhaustive reference lists, the authors provide focused lists of additional reading recommended to deepen understanding.

The resulting volume should provide you with a dynamic tour through the practice of pain neurosurgery, guided by some of the leading experts in North America. Additional volumes will cover each subspecialty area of neurosurgery, using the same case-based approach and board review features.

Nathan R. Selden, MD, PhD
Campagna Professor and Chair
Department of Neurological Surgery
Oregon Health & Science University

Contributors

Mandana A. Behbahani, MD
Department of Neurosurgery
University of Illinois at Chicago
Chicago, Illinois, USA

Sharona Ben-Haim, MD
Department of Neurosurgery
University of California
San Diego, CA

Marian M. Bercu, MD, MS
Center for Neuromodulation
Department of Neurosurgery, NYU Langone Medical Center
New York, NY

Jeffrey A. Brown, MD
Neurological Surgery
PC Lake Success
New York, NY

Edward Chang, MD
Department of Neurological Surgery
University of California
San Francisco, CA

Nauman S. Chaudhry, MD
Department of Neurosurgery
University of Illinois at Chicago
Chicago, Illinois, USA

Cletus Cheyuo, MD, PhD
Department of Neurosurgery
West Virginia University School of Medicine
Morgantown, WV

Daniel R. Cleary, MD, PhD
Department of Neurological Surgery
University of California-San Diego
San Diego, CA

Claire Collison, MS
Department of Neuroscience and Experimental Therapeutics
Albany Medical College
Albany, NY

Nicholas C. Field, MD
Department of Neurosurgery
Albany Medical College
Albany, NY

Brian J. A. Gill, MD
Department of Neurosurgery
Columbia University
New York, NY

Patrick J. Hunt
Medical Scientist Training Program
Baylor College of Medicine
Houston, TX

Roy S. Hwang, MD, MS
Department of Neurosurgery
Albany Medical College
Albany, NY

Patrick J. Karas, MD
Department of Neurosurgery
Baylor College of Medicine
Houston, TX

Farhan A. Khan
Department of Neurosurgery
Columbia University
New York, NY

Anthony Lee, PhD
University of California
San Francisco, CA

Emily Lehmann Levin, MD
Department of Neurosurgery
Michigan Medicine,
University of Michigan
Ann Arbor, MI

Alon Y. Mogilner, MD, PhD
Center for Neuromodulation,
Department of Neurosurgery
NYU Langone Medical Center
New York, NY

Innocent Njoku, MD
Department of Neurosurgery
Albany Medical College
Albany, NY

Julie G. Pilitsis, MD, PhD
Department of Neurosurgery
Albany Medical College
Albany, NY
Department of Neuroscience and
Experimental Therapeutics
Albany Medical College
Albany, NY

Ahmed M. Raslan, MD
Department of Neurological Surgery
Oregon Health & Science University
Portland, OR

Kunal Raygor, MD
Department of Neurological Surgery
University of California
San Francisco, CA

Sebastian Rubino, MD
Department of Neurosurgery
Albany Medical Center
Albany, NY

Shelby Sabourin, HSD
Department of Neurosciences and
Experimental Therapeutics
Albany Medical College
Albany, NY

Oren Sagher, MD
Department of Neurosurgery
Michigan Medicine,
University of Michigan
Ann Arbor, MI

Timothy Shepherd, MD, PhD
Department of Radiology
NYU Langone Medical Center
New York, NY

Sameer A. Sheth, MD, PhD
Department of Neurosurgery
Baylor College of Medicine
Houston, TX

Konstantin V. Slavin, MD
Department of Neurosurgery
University of Illinois at Chicago
Chicago, Illinois, USA

Zoe Teton, BS
Department of Neurological Surgery
Oregon Health & Science University
Portland, OR

Ashwin Viswanathan, MD
Department of Neurosurgery
Baylor College of Medicine
Houston, TX

Richard L. Weiner, MD, FACS, FAANS
Dallas Neurosurgical and Spine Associates
Department of Neurosurgery
University of Texas, Southwestern
Medical School
Dallas, TX

Christopher J. Winfree, MD
Department of Neurosurgery
Columbia University
New York, NY

Idiopathic Trigeminal Neuralgia in the Healthy Patient

Oren Sagher

1

Case Presentation

A 46-year-old woman presents to the clinic with a 10-year history of pain in the left side of the face. The pain is both in the forehead and the cheek. It is described by the patient as lancinating and like an electrical jolt. It occurs spontaneously, although it may also be triggered by wiping of the nose, touch, wind, and the brushing of teeth. The pain is episodic, and the patient is pain-free between episodes. The patient describes the initial onset of this pain 5 years prior as spontaneous and without inciting event. The initial occurrence of pain lasted only a week and was followed by a months' long remission. Since then, the patient has had several recurrences of her pain, each remitting several weeks later. She does state that the painful episodes have become longer and more intense with time, and that the remissions have not been completely pain-free more recently. After ineffective attempts to treat her condition with mild narcotic pain medications, she started taking Tegretol recently. This treated her pain effectively, but she has not been able to tolerate this medication due to granulocytopenia. Attempted treatment with baclofen and Neurontin has not been effective. Detailed neurological examination, including a full cranial nerve examination, is completely normal. Her eye and face appear normal, with a normal oral examination as well.

Questions

1. What is the likely diagnosis?
2. What diagnoses are important to exclude?
3. What is the most appropriate imaging modality?
4. What is the appropriate timing of further workup?

Assessment and Planning

The neurosurgeon suspects the diagnosis of trigeminal neuralgia. The lancinating nature of the pain, its trigeminal distribution, the presence of spontaneous remissions and recurrences, and the response to Tegretol are all hallmarks of this condition. It is important to note that trigeminal neuralgia is a rather uncommon cause of facial pain, accounting for approximately 10% of cases. It is therefore important to exclude other potential causes of trigeminal-distribution pain. These include such conditions as post-traumatic trigeminal neuropathy (such as post-dental procedure pain), atypical facial pain (in which pain frequently goes outside the trigeminal distribution), and trigeminal autonomic cephalgia (a condition related to cluster headache that is accompanied by conjunctival injection, tearing, and rhinorrhea). Usually, the description of the pain or the history of its evolution is of significant value in excluding these trigeminal neuralgia look-alikes.

Since the diagnosis of trigeminal neuralgia is a clinical one, based upon the history and examination, the role of imaging is mainly in excluding conditions that cause so-called secondary or provoked trigeminal neuralgia. Whereas idiopathic trigeminal neuralgia has, by definition, no overt cause, the secondary trigeminal neuralgias are usually related either to mass lesions around the trigeminal nerve (such as tumors in the cerebellopontine angle) or demyelination of the central nervous system (such as multiple sclerosis). In addition to excluding the presence of inciting pathology, brain magnetic resonance imaging (MRI) may also allow the neurosurgeon to get detailed images of the root entry zone of the trigeminal nerve. These images are usually obtained in specialized sequences that accentuate the signal differences between cerebral spinal fluid (CSF), nerves, and blood vessels, allowing the neurosurgeon to appreciate the presence of a vascular loop causing compression of the trigeminal nerve at the root entry zone. The addition of time-of-flight source images of a magnetic resonance angiogram (MRA) can provide further anatomical information on the nature of the neurovascular contact.

Oral Boards Review—Diagnostic Pearls

1. Trigeminal neuralgia is a clinical diagnosis, based on the description of the pain, its distribution, and the history of its evolution. It is not a radiographic diagnosis, and the use of MRI is strictly adjunct in the assessment and planning of treatment.
2. The description of trigeminal neuralgia pain by patients is incredibly stereotyped. Deviation from description of lancinating, episodic pain should be regarded as a "red flag" that trigeminal neuralgia may not be the correct diagnosis.
3. The physical examination of the patient with untreated trigeminal neuralgia is invariably normal. Any trigeminal deficits (e.g., numbness, jaw weakness) should raise concern for lesional or secondary pain conditions.
4. Although the initial bouts of trigeminal neuralgia give way to pain-free remissions, with time, these remissions may not be strictly pain-free. Many patients develop a constant, frequently burning, component of facial pain that may persist after the lancinating pain has resolved. Such constant pain has been termed trigeminal neuralgia, type 2 (Type 2 TN) in counter-distinction to the lancinating pain, known as trigeminal neuralgia, type 1 (Type 1 TN). Many patients eventually come to have both Type 1 TN and Type 2 TN symptoms.

In the present case, the patient had classic features of Type 1 TN, with a more recent minor contribution of Type 2 TN symptoms. Her examination was consistent with a diagnosis of trigeminal neuralgia. A prior routine brain MRI excluded any

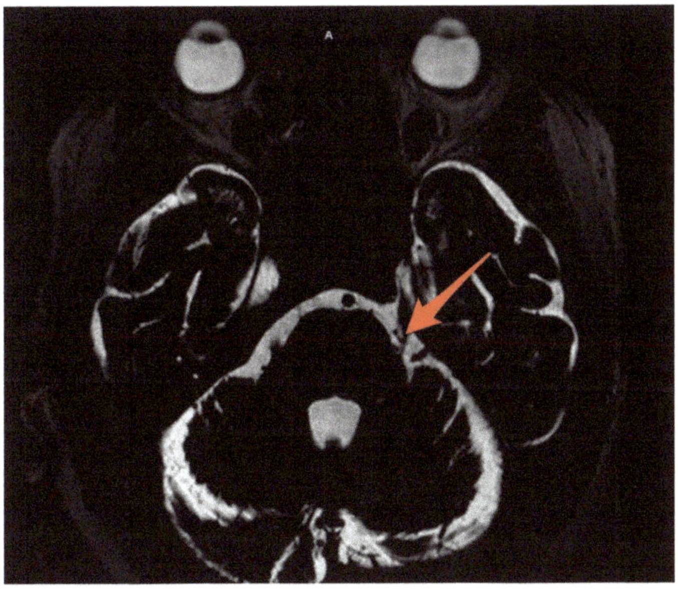

Figure 1.1. Thin-cut T2 MRI FIESTA sequence image demonstrating the typical appearance of neurovascular contact between a branch of the superior cerebellar artery and the trigeminal nerve entry zone on the left (arrow).

mass lesions around the trigeminal nerve, and the diagnosis of demyelinating disease was also discarded due to the lack of concordant history or any suggestive findings on her brain MRI. A high-definition MRI FIESTA (Fast Imaging Employing Steady-state Acquisition; termed CISS [Constructive Interference Steady State] on Siemens scanners) sequence showed a vascular loop making contact with the *left* trigeminal nerve at the root entry zone (Figure 1.1). This was confirmed by her MRA source images (Figure 1.2). Incidental note was made of a vascular loop making contact with the *right* trigeminal nerve as well.

Questions

1. How do these clinical and radiological findings influence surgical planning?
2. What is the significance of neurovascular contact contralateral to the patient's symptoms?
3. How would the absence of a neurovascular contact on the symptomatic side influence plans for surgery?

Decision Making

A history of unilateral, lancinating facial pain, with spontaneous remissions and recurrences and a response to Tegretol, is virtually diagnostic of trigeminal neuralgia. The absence of mass lesions along the trigeminal nerve means that the timing of surgical intervention would be strictly at the choice of the patient. If medical treatment is effective and well-tolerated, there is no reason to offer surgery to relieve symptoms, regardless of the presence of neurovascular compression. If the patient cannot tolerate

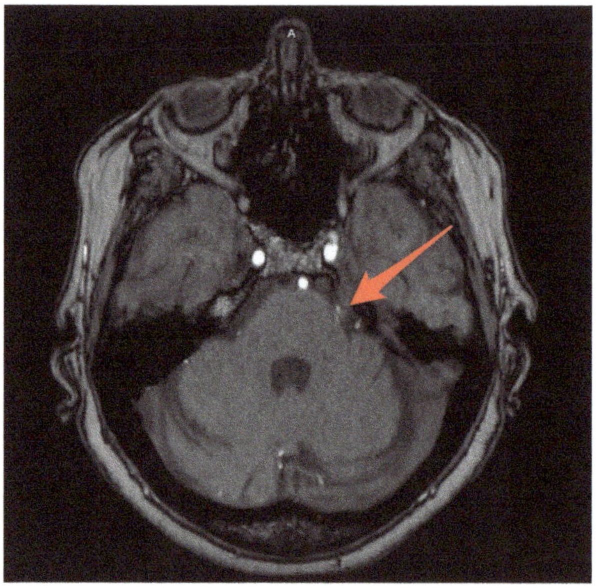

Figure 1.2. MR Angiography source image of the same region seen in Figure 1, demonstrating the vascular nature of the compressing structure at the root entry zone of the trigeminal nerve (arrow).

the medical treatment, or if medical treatment does not adequately control symptoms, however, surgery is indicated.

The choice of surgery for the treatment of idiopathic trigeminal neuralgia is complex and dependent on the surgeon's expertise and patient's preference. In general, however, patients who are young and healthy should be considered first for microvascular decompression (MVD) surgery, since it offers the most robust long-term results with the least risk of complications related to deafferentation. Other procedures for trigeminal neuralgia (outlined elsewhere in this book) all injure the trigeminal nerve to some extent and are subject to the risks related to such intentional nerve injury. In addition to age and health status, other factors that influence the choice of surgical procedure include the distribution of pain. Patients such as the one presented here, who have pain involving the ophthalmic (V1) division of the trigeminal nerve, are poor candidates for nerve-lesioning procedures that may put them at risk of corneal anesthesia, corneal exposure, and keratitis.

Questions

1. How does the absence of a convincing neurovascular contact on MRI influence MVD surgery?
2. What is the significance of neurovascular contact by a surface vein (rather than an artery)?

Surgical Procedure

MVD is a major procedure carried out under general anesthetic with a Foley catheter in place, IV access, and invasive arterial blood pressure monitoring. Brainstem auditory evoked responses (BAERs) are routinely used, as excessive retraction on the cerebellum to visualize the trigeminal nerve may put hearing at risk. Facial nerve monitoring and trigeminal nerve monitoring may also be performed.

Patients are positioned either semilateral or lateral, with the head in Mayfield pins turned to expose the retroauricular region. The head is usually tilted downward in order to improve the surgical angle to the trigeminal nerve. The ipsilateral shoulder is frequently taped down to improve the angle of visualization. The incision used may be "C" shaped, linear, or "S" shaped, but it should always span the asterion so that the angle of the transverse sinus and sigmoid sinus can be defined in the bony opening. This angle must be developed to allow the surgeon access to the upper portion of the cerebellopontine angle. Once the scalp is opened, the surgeon can perform either a craniotomy or a craniectomy, based on the sinus angle. The edges of the transverse and sigmoid sinuses should be seen after the bony removal is complete. The size of the cranial opening is variable, but it is usually around 3 cm in diameter. The mastoid air cells should be waxed. The dura is opened and CSF is allowed to drain, until the cerebellum relaxes and CSF spontaneously drains from the opening. At this point, the surgeon gently retracts the upper portion of the lateral cerebellar hemisphere, proceeding under high magnification along the junction of the tentorium and petrous face, until the petrosal vein comes into view. This vein, emanating from the superior petrosal sinus, is frequently sectioned, as it commonly obscures the trigeminal nerve deep to it. If it is possible to preserve all or part of this venous complex, the surgeon may choose to do so, but never at the expense of access to the trigeminal nerve. The trigeminal nerve is usually seen as a thick white band, surrounded by arachnoid membrane. It runs close to, but significantly deeper than, the facial/vestibular/cochlear complex that is frequently encountered first during the surgical approach. After freeing up the arachnoid adhesions around the trigeminal nerve, special attention is paid to the vessel abutting the nerve. If this vessel is an artery, it can be manipulated and mobilized away from the nerve, and a piece of Teflon felt can be interposed between them. If the compressive vessel proves to be a vein, it may not be possible to mobilize it. In such cases, the vein is coagulated and divided, in order to release any compression from the nerve.

Following the completion of the decompression, the dura is closed. The bone flap may be replaced or a bone substitute used, but this is not a necessity. The incision is closed tightly in layers to reduce the risk of CSF leak.

Oral Boards Review—Management Pearls

1. It is important to position the head with adequate turning so as to expose the retroauricular region and with a downward tilt of the head to improve the surgical angle.
2. BAER monitoring is useful to reduce the risk of hearing loss with surgery, as cerebellar retraction and manipulation in the vicinity of the trigeminal nerve may cause unrecognized stretching of the nearby cochlear fibers.
3. Sacrifice of the petrosal vein may be necessary in order to provide adequate access to the trigeminal nerve.
4. The trigeminal nerve is deeper and larger than the VII/VIII complex.

5. Infrequently, there is a tubercle of the petrous face directly over the trigeminal nerve that may partially obscure it from view. It is important to work around this visual obstruction and to resist temptation to drill it down, as it is usually the representation of an air cell in the temporal bone.
6. It is important to thoroughly inspect the trigeminal nerve before placing any interposing Teflon.
7. Arterial compression may occur anywhere along the trigeminal nerve, although it is most commonly seen in its rostral/ventral aspect.

Pivot Points

1. If a healthy patient presents with classic features of idiopathic Type 1 TN, that person should be considered first for a MVD.
2. Imaging does not play a role in the diagnosis of trigeminal neuralgia, except to exclude the possibility of secondary, or provoked, trigeminal neuralgia.
3. FIESTA (or CISS) MRA sequences on MRI inform the surgeon about the anatomy of the neurovascular compression, helping direct the surgeon's attention at the time of surgery.
4. BAER monitoring during surgery is an important safeguard against excessive retraction.

Aftercare

Patients are usually observed in an intensive care unit setting on the first night after surgery. They are mobilized as soon as possible, and are usually allowed to leave the hospital in short order. A short course of steroids is often prescribed to lessen the incidence of aseptic meningitis after surgery. Routine imaging is not necessary. Small pseudomeningoceles are not uncommon, and they usually resolve spontaneously.

Complications and Management

The most frequent complication of surgery is aseptic meningitis, probably related to blood in the CSF or the presence of Teflon. Symptoms consist of headache, neck stiffness, and low-grade fever. The usual treatment of these symptoms consists of a short burst of steroids. Of course, on the differential for such symptoms is septic meningitis. If the patient presents with such symptoms but appears more ill than expected, or does not respond to steroids, a lumbar puncture is indicated to rule out infection.

MVD may also be complicated by CSF rhinorrhea, usually related to CSF egress from the dural opening through a mastoid air cell into the middle ear and through the Eustachian tubes into the nasopharynx. When present, CSF rhinorrhea is relatively straightforward to manage, given the superficial nature of the CSF egress pathway. A lumbar drain may be placed temporarily to allow the hole in the mastoid air cell to seal, but if this does not resolve the issue, a superficial re-exploration, with resealing of the air cells, will stop the leak.

Less frequent complications include trigeminal sensory loss, hearing loss, facial paralysis, or cerebellar infarction. Despite the manipulation of the trigeminal nerve inherent in this surgery, appreciable sensory loss does not typically occur after MVD surgery unless the manipulation is significant. Hearing loss, on the other hand, may occur with far less manipulation or retraction, especially in older patients. BAER monitoring is helpful to reduce the risk of this complication. If waveforms diminish during the surgical approach, it is advisable to temporarily cease manipulation and retraction and allow waveforms to recover before continuing. Facial paralysis is very unusual, and it is usually a sign of excessive retraction. It is frequently accompanied by significant hearing loss. Cerebellar stroke is usually a sign of significant cerebellar retraction, or suboptimal positioning at the start of surgery. Some authors claim that sacrifice of the petrosal vein predisposes to cerebellar infarction, but this claim is controversial, with a recent study that specifically examined this issue that reported no increase in risk of cerebellar stroke.

Oral Boards Review—Complications Pearls

1. Careful patient positioning is essential to improve visualization and reduce the need for cerebellar retraction during surgery, thus reducing the risk of the most serious complications of the operation.
2. The most common complications of MVD surgery, aseptic meningitis and CSF rhinorrhea, are relatively straightforward to manage.
3. BAER monitoring allows the surgeon to reduce tension on the facial and cochlear nerves, reducing the risk of cranial neuropathies as a result of surgery.

Evidence and Outcomes

Numerous retrospective studies have documented the results of MVD surgery in the treatment of trigeminal neuralgia, although there are no prospective studies comparing its efficacy to other modalities of treatment. MVD is expected to provide relief of trigeminal neuralgia pain in 95–99% of patients immediately after surgery, but like other surgical approaches to this disease, longer-term outcomes demonstrate a time-dependent recurrence rate that is not insignificant. In the largest published trial of MVD surgery, over a long follow-up period, Dr. Jannetta's group published a 70% pain-free outcome at 10 years. This is a significantly better long-term result than other surgical approaches to trigeminal neuralgia, such as percutaneous lesioning procedures and stereotactic radiosurgery. These favorable long-term outcomes come at a price, however, as this operation does have a higher major morbidity and mortality rate than the other, less invasive options.

Further Reading

Barker, F. G., Jannetta, P. J., Bissonette, D. J., Larkins, M. V., & Jho, H. D. (1996). The long-term outcome of microvascular decompression for trigeminal neuralgia. *New England Journal of Medicine*, *334*(17), 1077–1083. http://doi.org/10.1056/NEJM199604253341701

Wang, D. D., Raygor, K. P., Cage, T. A., Ward, M. M., Westcott, S., Barbaro, N. M., & Chang, E. F. (2017). Prospective comparison of long-term pain relief rates after first-time microvascular decompression and stereotactic radiosurgery for trigeminal neuralgia. *Journal of Neurosurgery, 123*, 1–10. http://doi.org/10.3171/2016.9.JNS16149

Pathmanaban, O. N., O'Brien, F., Al-Tamimi, Y. Z., Hamerbeck-Ward, C. L., Rutherford, S. A., & King, A. T. (2017). Safety of superior petrosal vein sacrifice during microvascular decompression of the trigeminal nerve. *World Neurosurgery, 103*, 84–87. http://doi.org/10.1016/j.wneu.2017.03.117

Miller, J. P., Acar, F., & Burchiel, K. J. (2009). Classification of trigeminal neuralgia: clinical, therapeutic, and prognostic implications in a series of 144 patients undergoing microvascular decompression. *Journal of Neurosurgery, 111*(6), 1231–1234. http://doi.org/10.3171/2008.6.17604

Idiopathic Trigeminal Neuralgia in the Elderly

Kunal Raygor, Anthony Lee, and Edward Chang

2

Case Presentation

An 86-year-old man with a history of a cardiac pacemaker placed for atrial fibrillation presents to clinic with a 5-year history of right-sided, episodic, lancinating facial pain in the maxillary (V2) distribution, consistent with trigeminal neuralgia (TN). He has used carbamazepine with good pain relief for years; however, his pain broke through and he was started on oxcarbazepine and then lamotrigine. His partner has noticed worsening memory since starting the additional medications, and his labs have demonstrated hyponatremia. In addition to his arrhythmia, his medical history is significant for hypertension, hyperlipidemia, prostate adenocarcinoma without evidence of metastases, and poorly compensated congestive heart failure. On detailed neurologic examination, he has trouble remembering objects, but cranial nerve and strength exams are normal. MRI demonstrates a segment of the right superior cerebellar artery causing compression of the trigeminal nerve at the root-entry zone.

Questions

1. What medications are commonly used to treat type 1 TN?
2. What are the common side effects of those medications?

Treatment Options—Medical

Treatment of TN —both in the young and the elderly—includes medical and surgical approaches. Type 1 TN is typically treated with anticonvulsant medications, including carbamazepine (CBZ), oxcarbazepine (OXC), lamotrigine, gabapentin, and baclofen, with varying success. The American Academy of Neurology (AAN) and European Federation of Neurological Societies (EFNS) recommend both CBZ and OXC as first-line drugs for treatment of TN.[1] Patients unresponsive to these first-line medications can try an additional medication—including lamotrigine, gabapentin, and baclofen, to name a few—or should be referred for possible surgical intervention. Although the common side effects—memory loss, leucopenia, hyponatremia, and dermatologic reactions—can occur in all patients, they are especially concerning in the elderly, given cross-reactivity with other medications via the liver's cytochrome pathway. In particular, the elderly can be sensitive to CBZ because older patients have lower levels of non-glycated albumin, a major ligand of CBZ, which can lead to increased serum CBZ levels.[2] Unlike CBZ, OXC bypasses the cytochrome P-450 pathway and thus avoids many of the drug-drug interactions that affect the use of CBZ. In fact, Kutluay et al.[3] showed that OXC has been shown to be equally effective for patients over the age of 65 as for patients aged 18 to 64, without significant differences in adverse events. In their series, the incidence of nausea, dizziness, and somnolence was 17%, 17%, and 15%, respectively, in the elderly, compared to 20%, 29%, and 24% in the younger cohort. To help prevent significant side effects in elderly patients on anticonvulsants, it is recommended that those patients receive baseline measures of blood counts, electrolytes, liver function, and measures of bone metabolism.[4]

Questions

1. What ablative and non-ablative surgical options exist?
2. What are the common adverse effects of the surgical treatments for medically refractory TN?
3. What surgical option provides the longest duration of pain freedom?

Treatment Options—Surgical

Although medical treatment is the first-line for TN, surgical intervention is indicated for optimal pain relief in the setting of poor drug efficacy or severe side effects. Both ablative and non-ablative procedures have been used to treat medically refractory TN.

Ablative procedures include stereotactic radiosurgery (SRS) and percutaneous rhizolysis of the Gasserian ganglion via radiofrequency ablation (PRZ), glycerol injection (PGZ), or balloon compression (PBC). Microvascular decompression (MVD) is the standard non-ablative procedure for TN. The three percutaneous procedures are effective at providing immediate pain relief, with 98.6% and 100% of elderly patients receiving PBC and PRZ, respectively, obtaining complete pain relief at the time of discharge from the hospital.[5,6] Unfortunately, the pain relief after these procedures is typically short-lived, with ~25–50% of patients developing pain recurrence by 3 years post-procedure.[5] In addition, patients can develop sensory loss and even painful dysesthesias or anesthesia dolorosa after these ablative procedures with one study reporting 37% of patients developing sensory loss at a median 7.5 months follow-up after PGZ.[7] When performing these percutaneous procedures, surgeons and anesthesiologists should be aware of the trigeminal-cardiac reflex, as sudden spikes in blood pressure or cardiac arrhythmias may occur. Stereotactic radiosurgery (SRS) is the final major ablative procedure used to treat medically refractory TN. Because it requires no anesthesia, SRS should always be considered in the elderly who may have co-morbid conditions that limit their ability to receive anesthesia. SRS is typically performed with Gamma Knife or Cyberknife radiosurgery. When Gamma Knife is used, one or two 4 millimeter isocenters are used to target the cisternal portion of the trigeminal nerve with an average initial dose of 80 Gy. SRS leads to delayed pain relief as opposed to the other ablative procedures, with onset of pain relief usually occurring 4–8 weeks after radiosurgery. A recent study showed that SRS in patients >70 years of age led to a favorable outcome (complete or significant but incomplete pain relief with or without medications) in 82% of patients at 1 year, 60% at 3 years, and 38% at 5 years, with 17% of patients developing some type of sensory deficit.[8] It is likely that age does not significantly impact the success of SRS based on multivariate analyses[9] though a prior study has shown that early SRS is more effective than late SRS at providing pain control[10]. Much like the other ablative procedures, SRS commonly leads to sensory loss—in fact, sensory loss is predictive of pain freedom after SRS[9]—and can also cause painful dysesthesias or anesthesia dolorosa.

Though ablative strategies do work for many patients, they tend to provide less durable pain relief than the non-ablative strategy—microvascular decompression (MVD). Operative microvascular decompression has been shown to have a longer duration of pain freedom than SRS as an initial treatment modality for medically refractory TN in patients of all ages.[9] In the elderly, multiple studies have shown that MVD is as effective as it is in younger patients, with an equivalent rate of complications.[11–15] The most common complications after a retrosigmoid craniotomy or craniectomy for microvascular decompression of the trigeminal nerve are cerebrospinal fluid (CSF) leak or pseudomeningocele, which occur in about 7% of patients, and wound infections which occur in up to 4% of patients.[9] Less common complications include aseptic meningitis, postoperative hematoma or ischemic infarct, and injury to the seventh or eighth cranial nerves. Unfortunately, patient co-morbidities are not standardized or controlled for in most of these studies; however, in our practice, we have found that if a patient is deemed safe to receive general anesthesia, we tend to recommend MVD as the initial treatment modality given its relative safety and superior effectiveness. We also recommend against ablative procedures for patients with TN symptoms in the ophthalmic (V1) distribution due to the risk of keratitis. Oh et al.[13] demonstrated that in a small population of 27 patients >65 years old receiving MVD and 18 receiving SRS, those that underwent MVD had a longer duration of pain freedom, which is consistent with a recent report of patients of all ages undergoing first-time MVD or SRS.[9] Nevertheless, studies that directly compare MVD and SRS in the elderly with larger sample sizes and prospectively collected data are lacking.

Oral Boards Review—Therapeutic Pearls

1. Medications are the first line of treatment for idiopathic TN in the elderly, with first-line drugs including CBZ and OXC. In patients taking multiple medications, OXC may be preferred due to fewer drug-drug interactions.
2. Surgical approaches should be considered in patients with poor pain control despite numerous medications or in those with intolerable side effects.
3. Ablative procedures include stereotactic radiosurgery and percutaneous rhizolysis of the Gasserian ganglion via radiofrequency ablation (PRZ), glycerol injection (PGZ), or balloon compression (PBC). All ablative procedures tend to cause sensory changes and have limited duration of pain control. SRS is the least invasive of these procedures, but the onset of pain relief tends to be 4–8 weeks after radiosurgery.
4. Microvascular decompression (MVD) is the sole non-ablative procedure for refractory TN. Despite being the most invasive option, MVD offers the longest duration of pain freedom in multiple studies and is as effective in the elderly as it is in younger patients with a similar risk profile.

In the present case, the patient has multiple medical co-morbidities but also has persistent medically refractory trigeminal pain. Given his concurrent medical issues, he is recommended to undergo noninvasive stereotactic radiosurgery, which is the least invasive surgical option and provides equivalent pain control compared to the other ablative options.

Further Reading

1. Cruccu G, Gronseth G, Alksne J, et al. AAN-EFNS guidelines on trigeminal neuralgia management. *Eur J Neurol.* 2008;15(10):1013–1028.
2. Koyama H, Sugioka N, Uno A, Mori S, Nakajima K. Age-related alteration of carbamazepine-serum protein binding in man. *J Pharm Pharmacol.* 1999;51(9):1009–1014.
3. Kutluay E, McCague K, D'Souza J, Beydoun A. Safety and tolerability of oxcarbazepine in elderly patients with epilepsy. *Epilepsy Behav.* 2003;4(2):175–180.
4. Oomens M, Forouzanfar T. Pharmaceutical management of trigeminal neuralgia in the elderly. *Drugs Aging.* 2015;32(9):717–726.
5. Tang Y, Jin D, Bian J, Li X, Lai G, Ni J. Long-term outcome of computed tomography-guided percutaneous radiofrequency thermocoagulation for classic trigeminal neuralgia patients older than 70 years. *J Craniofac Surg.* 2014;25(4):1292–1295.
6. Ying X, Wang H, Deng S, Chen Y, Zhang J, Yu W. Long-term outcome of percutaneous balloon compression for trigeminal neuralgia patients elder than 80 years: A STROBE-compliant article. *Medicine (Baltimore).* 2017;96(39):e8199.
7. Lunsford LD. Treatment of tic douloureux by percutaneous retrogasserian glycerol injection. *JAMA.* 1982;248(4):449–453.
8. Cohen J, Mousavi SH, Faraji AH, et al. Stereotactic radiosurgery as initial surgical management for elderly patients with trigeminal neuralgia. *Stereotact Funct Neurosurg.* 2017;95(3):158–165.
9. Wang DD, Raygor KP, Cage TA, et al. Prospective comparison of long-term pain relief rates after first-time microvascular decompression and stereotactic radiosurgery for trigeminal neuralgia. *J Neurosurg.* 2018;128(1):68–77.
10. Mousavi SH, Niranjan A, Huang MJ, et al. Early radiosurgery provides superior pain relief for trigeminal neuralgia patients. *Neurology.* 2015;85(24):2159–2165.
11. Ferroli P, Acerbi F, Tomei M, Tringali G, Franzini A, Broggi G. Advanced age as a contraindication to microvascular decompression for drug-resistant trigeminal neuralgia: Evidence of prejudice? *Neurol Sci.* 2010;31(1):23–28.
12. Günther T, Gerganov VM, Stieglitz L, Ludemann W, Samii A, Samii M. Microvascular decompression for trigeminal neuralgia in the elderly: Long-term treatment outcome and comparison with younger patients. *Neurosurgery.* 2009;65(3):482; discussion 482.
13. Oh IH, Choi SK, Park BJ, Kim TS, Rhee BA, Lim YJ. The treatment outcome of elderly patients with idiopathic trigeminal neuralgia: Micro-vascular decompression versus gamma knife radiosurgery. *J Korean Neurosurg Soc.* 2008;44(4):199–204.
14. Sekula RF, Marchan EM, Fletcher LH, Casey KF, Jannetta PJ. Microvascular decompression for trigeminal neuralgia in elderly patients. *J Neurosurg.* 2008;108(4):689–691.
15. Sekula RF, Frederickson AM, Jannetta PJ, Quigley MR, Aziz KM, Arnone GD. Microvascular decompression for elderly patients with trigeminal neuralgia: A prospective study and systematic review with meta-analysis. *J Neurosurg.* 2011;114(1):172–179.

Secondary Trigeminal Neuralgia (Balloon Compression Rhizolysis)

Jeffrey A. Brown

3

Case Presentation

A 56-year-old woman presents with an 18-month history of stabbing right jaw pain that began when she was drying her face. On a McGill Pain Questionnaire she selected the descriptives *shooting, stabbing, sharp, terrifying, unbearable, torturing*, and *excruciating* to describe the nature of her pain. Fifteen years ago she had an episode of right facial numbness that resolved. She was diagnosed with multiple sclerosis (MS). She has had a thyroid nodule excised and a partial thyroidectomy. She has chronic low back pain for which she has been treated with physical therapy, facet blocks, and epidural steroids. Current medications are gabapentin 300 mg three times daily, baclofen 20 mg three times daily, clonazepam 1mg three times daily, levothyroxine 100 mcg daily, bupropion 150 mg daily, fluoxetine 20 mg daily, and hydrocodone prn.

On examination, her facial sensation is intact to cold temperature, light touch, and pinprick in all three divisions. She has normal muscle tone, coordination, strength, and gait.

Questions

1. What is the likely diagnosis?
2. What is the most appropriate imaging modality?
3. What anatomical areas should be appropriately reviewed and why?

Assessment and Planning

The neurosurgeon suspects a diagnosis of trigeminal neuralgia. Given the history of multiple sclerosis, he believes that the neuralgia is secondary to the multiple sclerosis. However, the patient has had no documented active episodes of MS since the single episode of numbness more than a decade ago, and those symptoms all resolved. She had no pain at the time of that episode.

Current accepted terminology divides the condition into three subclasses. A patient with trigeminal neuralgia type 1 (TN1) has the better-known entity of idiopathic, spontaneous facial pain that is predominantly episodic intermittent, characterized as electrical shocks or stabs precipitated by touching the face, speaking, eating, swallowing, or by a cool breeze blowing across the face. A patient with trigeminal neuralgia type 2 (TN2) has an element of constant, usually described as burning, pain. Trigeminal deafferentation pain is a consequence of ablative treatment for TN. A patient with atypical facial pain has an associated somatoform pain disorder. The category of symptomatic TN is reserved for patients with MS.

The most appropriate imaging modality when treating a patient with suspected trigeminal neuralgia is an MRI scan. It should then be possible to determine whether there is a vascular association with the trigeminal nerve, an associated tumor, or the plaques of multiple sclerosis. An adequate study requires a separate sequence that is not routinely performed. The sequence is called by the acronym FIESTA (fast imaging employing steady state acquisition cycled phases) with a machine manufactured by General Electric; with a Siemens machine, it is called by the acronym CISS (constructive interference with steady state gradient-echo sequence.) When combined with thin slices, these sequences distinguish cerebrospinal fluid, cranial nerves and associated pre pontine cisternal vessels. Note, if there has been a previous microvascular decompression (MVD), imaging of the nerve may be difficult.

Trigeminal neuralgia is well known to be associated with MS. FLAIR or T2 sequences are best used to detect evidence for a diagnosis of MS. While the MRI can be diagnostic of MS, it is still conceivable that the cause of the facial pain is vascular compression and not multiple sclerosis. If there are plaques seen within the brainstem along the trigeminal pathways, then MS is more likely to be the cause.

Rarely, a parotid gland tumor may cause dysesthetic, continuous, burning neuropathic facial pain. It is important to that the evaluative MRI for trigeminal neuropathic pain visualizes the skull base and the parotid gland, as well as the trigeminal nerve and brainstem.

Decision Making

This is a healthy woman with a history of the onset of MS 15 years previously, with no evidence of progression of her disease, who has the recent onset of trigeminal neuropathic pain. It is known that MS is associated with trigeminal neuropathic pain, but why has the pain emerged at this point when there is no evidence to suggest progression of MS? Dr. Peter Jannetta established the relationship of arterial and venous compression with the pain of trigeminal neuralgia. Beginning with his first modern microvascular decompression of the trigeminal nerve, done in 1966 and reported in a series of patients in 1967, he, along with others, clarified that vascular compression leads to dysmyelinization within the nerve. Jannetta advocated that the Vth nerve contained a cone of central fiber myelin that extended into the cisternal portion of the nerve. This central myelin that was manufactured by oligodendroglial cells was distinct from peripheral myelin that was manufactured by Schwann cells. The central myelin was hypothesized to be more sensitive to injury. Trigeminal compression in the root entry zone is a cause of short circuits (ephaptic transmission) in the nerve that translate as the pain of trigeminal neuralgia. Clinical experience has shown, however, that compression anywhere along the cisternal portion of the trigeminal nerve can cause trigeminal neuropathic pain.

Assessment and Planning

In this patient, a FIESTA MRI shows a vascular association with the medial mid cisternal portion of the right trigeminal nerve at the level of the pons (Figure 3.1). However, the T2 weighted images show a sclerotic plaque in the brainstem (Figure 3.2).

The plaque in this patient is associated with the primary sensory nucleus of the trigeminal nerve, which explains the symptomatic onset of ipsilateral sensory loss 15 years ago. The plaque does not enhance, suggesting that the onset of neuropathic pain is not related to an acute MS lesion.

> **Question**
>
> 1. Is it possible for a patient with MS to develop trigeminal neuropathic pain unrelated to the MS, and will the patient respond to a microvascular decompression?

Decision Making

In this case, because the MRI showed contact of the nerve with a vessel, but not distortion, and the brainstem lesion was adjacent to the trigeminal pathway, the neurosurgeon elected to proceed with an ablative procedure.

Current practice includes several options for ablative trigeminal surgery. In historical order, they are

1. Partial sensory rhizotomy
2. Radiofrequency thermal rhizotomy
3. Glycerol rhizotomy
4. Gamma knife radiosurgery
5. Percutaneous balloon compression
6. Cyberknife radiosurgery

Comprehensive review of the results of treatment among these modalities over many years shows that the outcomes are similar and no single treatment is clearly superior to

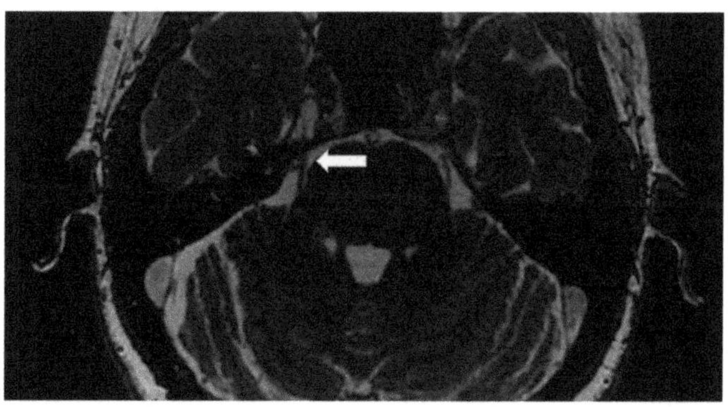

Figure 3.1. Axial MRI with FIESTA technique. Arrow points to the intracisternal portion of the right trigeminal nerve with a distal vascular association present.

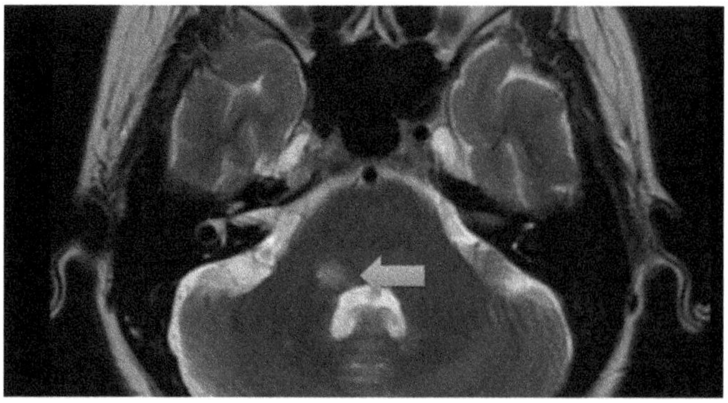

Figure 3.2. Axial MRI with T2 weighting. Arrow points to a sclerotic plaque in the brainstem in proximity to the primary trigeminal sensory nucleus.

the other. The choice of the ablative procedure should be tailored to the needs of the patient.

Elderly patients may require blood thinners for maintenance of cardiac stents or for cardiac arrhythmias. If it is determined that the anticoagulant should not be discontinued, the best option may be radiosurgery with the gamma knife. No invasive element is needed in this case, only application of cranial frame. Cyberknife radiosurgery requires a spinal tap and cisternography. The treatment planning makes use of the CT coordinates of the skull and trigeminal nerve. Also, elderly patients may not be able to appropriately cooperate with the neurosurgeon to communicate the locus of intraoperative stimulation and sensory loss during thermal rhizotomy when awakening from propofol anesthetic. In the past, Brevitol anesthetic, when used by an experienced anesthetist, could be titrated for rapid recovery from the sedative dose used during lesion generation. Brevitol is no longer available. Recovery from propofol is not as quick, and the procedure is prolonged as a consequence.

A study of quality of life after treatment for trigeminal neuralgia showed that the best quality is achieved after a patient undergoes microvascular decompression. Among the ablative procedures, percutaneous balloon compression provided the best life quality.

In this case, the neurosurgeon and the patient elected to proceed with percutaneous balloon compression since medical treatment was no longer adequately effective.

The decision to proceed with any surgical procedure for trigeminal neuralgia depends on having completed an adequate trial of medical therapy with anticonvulsant medication. The dosage should be gradually titrated upward, since too high an initial dose will cause excessive sedation. The dose should be gradually increased until pain is controlled or the sedative effects of the medication are no longer tolerated. Side effects of anticonvulsant medication include difficulty with balance, memory, and concentration. Rarely, allergic side effects occur early on during treatment. There is no standard dose, and progression to multiple anticonvulsant drugs is unlikely to be beneficial.

What Are the Risks and Benefits of Balloon Compression?

Balloon compression has a higher incidence of masseter and pterygoid muscle weakness than other procedures (24%). This usually resolves within one month and may be associated with temporomandibular jaw discomfort because of muscular imbalance. Mild numbness is anticipated (83%) but with a low incidence of painful dysesthesias (4%).

Surgical Procedure

The procedure is done under general anesthesia using either an endotracheal tube or laryngeal mask airway. The patient need not cooperate for localization. Patients with MS should be premedicated with IV steroids in addition to single dose antibiotics. Aspirin used for anticoagulation should be discontinued in advance of the procedure as should any other oral anticoagulant. The procedure should only be done after imaging of the trigeminal nerve either by appropriate MRI or by CT scanning. Either the operating room and intraoperative fluoroscopy are used or biplane fluoroscopy in the angiography suite. Some neurosurgeons use the Axiom neuronavigation system to identify the foramen ovale. However, fluoroscopy is needed to identify the porous trigeminous, which is the target for the balloon tip.

Three fluoroscopic views are used. The cannula is larger than the #22 gauge spinal needle used with glycerol or thermal rhizotomy, so it is advisable to visualize the foramen ovale directly with a modified submental view (Figure 3.3). Initial direction of the cannula makes use of standard Haertel guidelines and a lateral fluoroscopic image to direct the cannula toward the radiographic intersection of clivus and petrous bone.

Note that the cannula remains extracranial and only the balloon catheter penetrates the intracranial interdural space. The balloon catheter is a #4 Fogarty embolectomy catheter (Edwards Lifesciences, Irvine, CA). The catheter tip is directed toward the dip in the petrous bone representing the porous trigeminous. This is seen by aligning the fluoro unit so as to position the ipsilateral petrous bone in the midpoint of the orbit radiographically (Figure 3.4). For V3 pain the catheter is positioned along the skull base and within the lateral portion of the porous. For V2 pain the catheter is positioned in

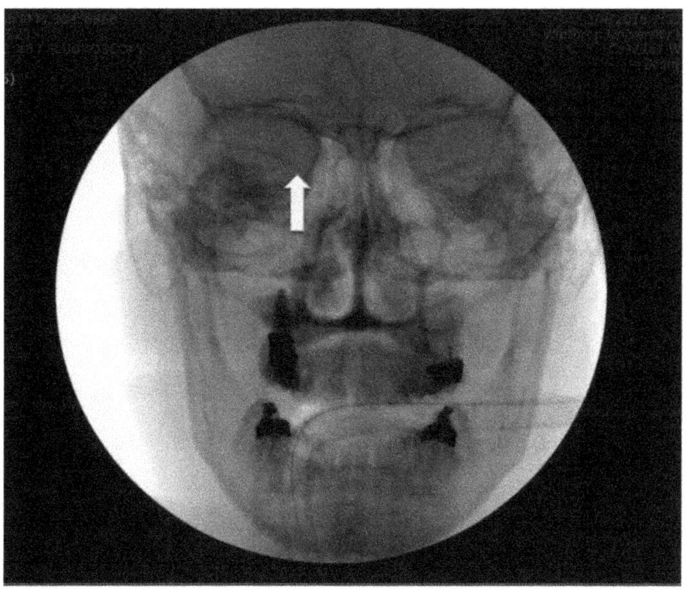

Figure 3.3. Modified submental view of the skull. The #14 gauge cannula has engaged the right foramen ovale. An inner stylet just penetrates it.

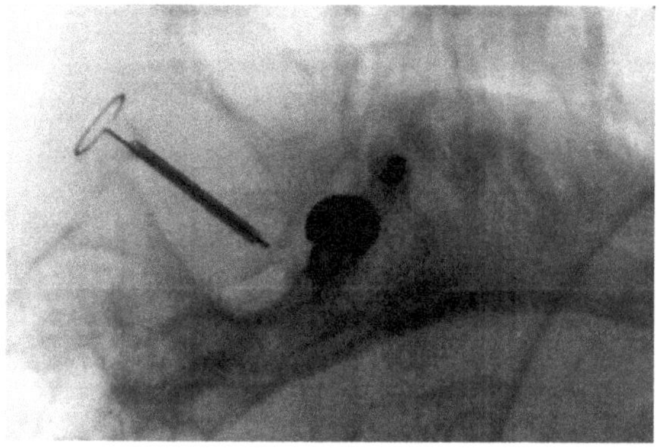

Figure 3.4. Modified anterior-posterior view of the skull with the dip in the petrous bone representing the porous trigeminous, the entrance to Meckel's cave, positioned in the center of the orbit radiographically (arrow).

the midpoint of the dip, and for V1 pain in the medial portion. Because Meckel's cave is angled medially, the catheter is positioned deeper for V1 pain than for V2 or V3. In each case the tip of the catheter should be set 1–2 mm beyond the edge of petrous ridge when the modified AP is used to visualize the porous. While the balloon is inflated, repeated lateral views are used to determine whether the required "pear" shape has been obtained (Figure 3.5).

Note that balloon compression is not trigeminal ganglion compression. It is compression of the retrogasserian trigeminal nerve within the confines of the porous trigeminous. This space is bordered by the petrous bone and the firm edge of the tentorial dura. The dura splits to allow passage of the trigeminal nerve into the

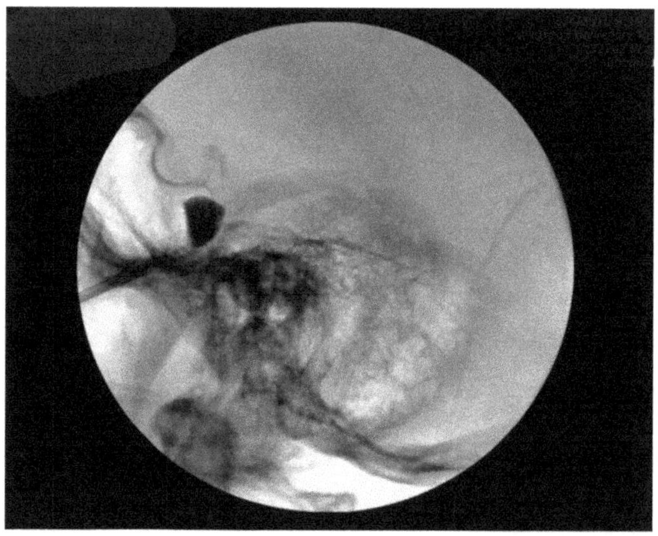

Figure 3.5. Lateral fluoroscopic image of the skull obtained during compression of the trigeminal nerve. The balloon has the typical "pear" shape indicating that its tip lies within the porous trigeminous, the entrance to Meckel's cave, in which the nerve is compressed against the skull base and the sharp edge of the dura.

posterior fossa. The "pear" represents the tip of the otherwise oval shaped balloon that lies within that space.

If the cannula is allowed to pass intracranially, then it may not be possible to inflate the balloon in the appropriate location, since the balloon must fully pass beyond the tip of the cannula.

Some neurosurgeons use a tuberculin syringe to inflate the balloon with 0.7 cc omnipaque or enough dye to obtain the "pear." The treating neurosurgeon in this case used an insoufflation syringe and digital pressure monitor to achieve an intraluminal pressure of 1.5 atm. Depending on the severity of the patient's pain the duration of compression is from one to three minutes.

During compression the neurosurgeon must be prepared for the trigeminal depressor response. This consists of brief bradycardia and hypotension. It can be blocked by preoperative placement of an external pacemaker programmed to respond should the heart rate drop below 40 beats/minute. In addition the anesthesiologist should be prepared to inject IV atropine.

In some cases a dumbbell shape is seen. This occurs when the catheter is positioned beyond the porous into the posterior fossa. The catheter should be withdrawn and repositioned should this occur. If a pear is not obtained and the balloon appears oval shaped on imaging, then the catheter must be advanced and repositioned so that its tip lies within the porous trigeminous. If bradycardia persists during compression, then the anesthesiologist should proceed to inject IV atropine. Should the foramen ovale not be seen with fluoroscopy, then a formal X-ray should be taken to best demonstrate it.

This patient underwent 1 ¼ minutes of compression to a pressure of 1.5 atmospheres and was discharged home from the post anesthesia recovery room four hours later.

Oral Boards Review—Management Pearls

1. The retrogasserian portion of the trigeminal nerve that lies within the porous trigeminous is the surgical target in balloon compression—not the ganglion.
2. The presence of a "pear shape" indicating compression within the porous is associated with successful pain relief. To confirm appropriate catheter position, a modified AP fluoroscopic image of the skull, with the petrous bone seen through the orbit, will show the dip in the petrous bone that represents the entrance to the posterior fossa for the trigeminal nerve.
3. The surgeon should be prepared for a "trigeminal depressor response" consisting of brief bradycardia and hypotension during compression of the trigeminal nerve.
4. The #14-gauge cannula used to introduce the balloon catheter engages the foramen ovale but should not penetrate beyond it.
5. A patient with an ipsilateral petrous ridge meningioma or acoustic neuroma and trigeminal neuralgia may still be treated by balloon compression, if the only symptoms are of severe trigeminal neuralgia and open surgery is a relative contraindication.

Pivot Points

1. The presence of a predominance of constant, burning, dysesthetic facial pain in the targeted dermatome is a contraindication to percutaneous balloon compression.
2. It must be medically possible to discontinue/reverse anticoagulation therapy, including aspirin, prior to and after compression for several days.
3. If a trigeminal tumor is present within Meckel's cave, balloon compression should not be performed since the balloon must traverse that area to reach the porous trigeminous.

Aftercare

The patient can be discharged home from the recovery room. Anticonvulsant medication should be tapered slowly over a period of weeks. Patients should be cautioned that if they develop aching pain in the preauricular jaw region, this can be treated with nonsteroidal agents or acetaminophen. It is a result of mal occlusion due to masseter and pterygoid muscle weakness.

Complications and Management

The status of the corneal reflex should be determined before discharging the patient. If the reflex is diminished, patients should begin using saline eye drops to protect from the effects of a dry cornea due to reduction in tearing associated with trigeminal injury. If the patient complains of severe eye pain, it may occur because of a corneal abrasion. If the eye grounds are red, then this is likely. A formal ophthalmologic exam and antibiotic eye drops are required.

What If the Trigeminal Pain Persists or Is Aggravated by the Procedure?

This can occur if the compression is mild. A period of up to one week may be needed before the pain resolves. Laboratory studies in rabbits have shown that there is ongoing inflammatory injury that occurs for days after the compression.

A few patients have developed diplopia. This also should resolve within a few days. Severe headache can occur from the chemical meningitis of mild subarachnoid hemorrhage. This can be seen on CT scan and treated with IV steroids until resolution.

If pain relief does not occur and the procedure did not engender numbness, then it can be repeated and the compression intensified by increasing the duration of compression.

Oral Boards Review—Complications Pearls

1. One should confirm the presence of the corneal reflex post procedure. If it is reduced, then the patient is at risk of a corneal abrasion or visual disturbance from reduced tearing.

2. Severe, constant eye pain associated with engorged, red eye grounds after the procedure most likely indicates that a corneal abrasion has occurred. This should be treated with antibiotic eye drops.
3. Jaw pain and tenderness post procedure is likely a consequence of mal occlusion from weakening of the ipsilateral masseter and pterygoid muscles. It can be alleviated by anti-inflammatory oral medication.
4. Severe post-operative headache and confusion may indicate the presence of sub-arachnoid hemorrhage. A CT scan is indicated and the headache will improve with steroids.

Evidence and Outcomes

In a series of 10 patients with MS who underwent MVD and in whom proven vascular compression was adequately treated, the actuarial pain free survival rate at three months was merely 50% and at two years it was reduced to only15%. In another study, Sindou, while reviewing his lifetime experience with trigeminal neuralgia, noted that those patients with vascular compression that caused distortion of the trigeminal nerve, as observed during surgery, had the best outcome.

Recurrence rates are considerably higher after balloon compression in patients with MS than in other patients. Studies specific to MS patients showed as high as a 50% recurrence rate in one year for one series and 86% at four years in another. Seventy percent of MS patients required more than one ablative procedure in that series.

Two weeks after the procedure this patient was reevaluated and her preoperative stabbing pain had resolved. On the McGill pain questionnaire her only descriptive was of incisional tenderness. She did not have detectable numbness to temperature, light touch, or pinprick in her face and was slowly tapering her anticonvulsant medications. Four months after the procedure the patient was pain free and off all medications.

Further Reading

1. Mullan S, Lichtor T. Percutaneous microcompression of the trigeminal ganglion for trigeminal neuralgia. *J Neurosurg.* 1983; 59(6):1007–1012.
2. Brown JA, Pilitsis JG. Percutaneous balloon compression for the treatment of trigeminal neuralgia: results in 56 patients based on balloon compression pressure monitoring. *Neurosurg Focus.* 2005; 18(5): E10.
3. Brown JA, Chittum CJ, Sabol D, Gouda JJ. Percutaneous balloon compression of the trigeminal nerve for treatment of trigeminal neuralgia. *Neurosurg Focus.* 1996; 1(2):e4; discussion 1 p following e4.
4. Alvarez-Pinzon AM, Wolf AL, Swedberg HN, et al. Comparison of percutaneous retrogasserian balloon compression and gamma knife radiosurgery for the treatment of trigeminal neuralgia in multiple sclerosis. *World Neurosurg.* 2017; 97: 590–594.
5. Martin S, Teo M, Suttner N. The effectiveness of percutaneous balloon compression in the treatment of trigeminal neuralgia in patients with multiple sclerosis. *J Neurosurg.* 2015; 123(6): 1507–1511.

6. Montano N, Papacci F, Cioni B, Di Bonaventura R, Meglio M. Percutaneous balloon compression for the treatment of trigeminal neuralgia in patients with multiple sclerosis. Analysis of the potentially prognostic factors. *Acta Neurochir (Wien).* 2012; 154(5): 779–783.
7. Leal PR, Hermier M, Froment JC, Souza MA, Cristino-Filho G, Sindou M. Preoperative demonstration of the neurovascular compression characteristics with special emphasis on the degree of compression, using high-resolution magnetic resonance imaging: a prospective study, with comparison to surgical findings, in 100 consecutive patients who underwent microvascular decompression for trigeminal neuralgia. *Acta Neurochir (Wien).* 2010; 152(5): 817–825.

Glossopharyngeal Neuralgia

Oren Sagher

4

Case Presentation

An 85-year-old man with a history of coronary artery disease, atrial fibrillation, and hypertension presents with a 5-year history of left neck, throat, and ear pain. It is described by the patient as lancinating and like an electrical jolt. It occurs spontaneously, although it is also triggered by swallowing. The pain is episodic, and the patient is pain-free between episodes. The patient describes the initial onset of this pain 5 years prior as spontaneous and without inciting event. The initial occurrence of pain resolved spontaneously and did not recur for the next several years. About one month before presentation, he began to experience similar attacks, which have increased in intensity and frequency since then. He has also experienced syncopal episodes with some of these attacks and was eventually implanted with a pacemaker. The attacks have continued to crescendo, and he has been unable to eat or drink for the last several days due to the pain. He was started on Tegretol, with some improvement, but began to experience sedation related to this medication. A detailed neurological examination, including a full cranial nerve examination, is completely normal. He has a normal oral examination as well.

Questions

1. What is the likely diagnosis?
2. What diagnoses are important to exclude?
3. What is the most appropriate imaging modality?
4. What is the appropriate timing of further work-up?

Assessment and Planning

The neurosurgeon suspects the diagnosis of glossopharyngeal neuralgia. The lancinating nature of the pain, its distribution, the presence of spontaneous remissions and recurrences, and the response to Tegretol are all hallmarks of this condition. Even in the absence of neurological deficits or obvious signs of malignancy on examination, it would be important to exclude the presence of a lesion with imaging of the head and neck. Deep ear pain may also be caused by geniculate neuralgia, but this is not typically associated with throat pain to the same extent as glossopharyngeal neuralgia.

The radiographic examination of choice in this case is an MRI. However, due to the existence of a pacemaker in this patient, an MRI could not be performed. In patients for whom MRI cannot be undertaken, CT imaging is usually sufficient. A thin-cut CT after administration of Omnipaque into the lumbar cistern can sometimes provide additional anatomical detail of the basal cisterns, but in this patient a regular CT was done, which did not disclose any lesions in the brain or brainstem, aside from a tortuous left vertebral artery (Figure 4.1). A CT of the neck was also normal.

Oral Boards Review—Diagnostic Pearls

1. Like trigeminal neuralgia, glossopharyngeal neuralgia is a clinical diagnosis, based on the description of the pain, its distribution, and the history of its evolution. It is not a radiographic diagnosis, and the use of imaging is strictly adjunct in the assessment and planning of treatment.
2. The description of glossopharyngeal neuralgia pain by patients is incredibly stereotyped.
3. Syncope is sometimes a component of the pain syndrome, and should strongly point the clinician toward this diagnosis.
4. The physical examination of the patient with untreated glossopharyngeal neuralgia is invariably normal. Any cranial nerve deficits should raise concern for lesional or secondary pain conditions.

In the present case, the patient had classic features of glossopharyngeal neuralgia, including the occurrence of syncopal episodes precipitated by swallowing. The imaging studies were reassuring for the absence of mass lesions in the head or neck, and there

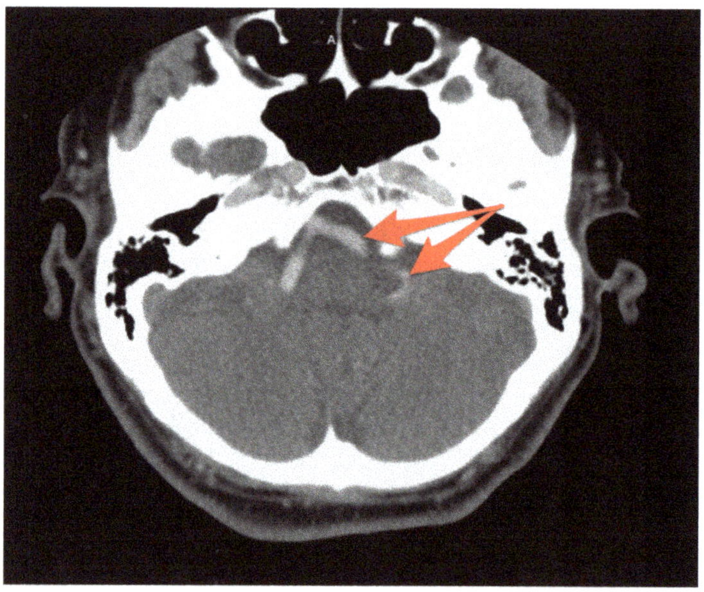

Figure 4.1. Thin-cut head CT angiography image, demonstrating an ectatic posterior vertebrobasilar junction, with a prominent loop of the posterior inferior cerebellar artery in the left cerebellomedullary angle (arrows). This distorted vascular anatomy may lead to compression of the glossopharyngeal nerve on the left, as it did in this patient.

was a suggestion of a vascular etiology, inasmuch as the patient had a tortuous vertebral artery on the symptomatic side.

Questions

1. How do these clinical and radiological findings influence surgical planning?
2. How does the age and health status of the patient influence surgical decision making?
3. How would the absence of a neurovascular contact on the symptomatic side influence plans for surgery?

Decision Making

A history of unilateral, lancinating ear and throat pain, with spontaneous remissions and recurrences, a response to Tegretol, and the presence of syncope are virtually diagnostic of glossopharyngeal neuralgia. If medical treatment is effective and well-tolerated, there is no reason to offer surgery to relieve symptoms. However, if the patient cannot tolerate the medical treatment (as happened in this case), or if medical treatment does not adequately control symptoms, surgery is indicated. In addition, when symptoms interfere with a patient's ability to eat and drink, surgical treatment should be performed expeditiously.

Unlike glossopharyngeal neuralgia's trigeminal counterpart, peripheral ablations are not easily performed. The co-location of the glossopharyngeal nerve with the vagus nerve and the jugular vein at the outlet of the nerve from the skull makes percutaneous ablation unfavorable. Lesioning of the glossopharyngeal nerve in isolation is, by and large, well tolerated, but it may cause significant swallowing problems and hoarseness if the vagus nerve is lesioned alongside it. The best surgical option for the treatment of glossopharyngeal neuralgia is therefore through exposure of the nerve in its intracranial segment. It is here where the surgeon has two options. The first option is a microvascular decompression (MVD) of the glossopharyngeal nerve from any obvious vascular loop making contact with the nerve near its root entry zone. The second option is a glossopharyngeal nerve section procedure. The latter operation, devised initially by Walter Dandy, is extremely well tolerated and has success rates that rival an MVD of the nerve. Moreover, the sectioning of the glossopharyngeal nerve requires far less manipulation of the neurovascular structures in the area and theoretically has a lower complication rate. Many surgeons prefer to defer the decision on which option to take until the time of surgery, allowing the operative findings to dictate whether an MVD is feasible or whether a section of the nerve would be preferable.

Questions

1. How does the absence of a convincing neurovascular contact on imaging influence MVD surgery?
2. How does the age and health of a patient influence surgical decision making?

Surgical Procedure

Microvascular decompression/glossopharyngeal nerve section is a major procedure carried out under general anesthetic with a Foley catheter in place, IV access, and invasive arterial blood pressure monitoring. Brainstem auditory evoked responses (BAERs) are routinely used. Facial nerve monitoring and trigeminal nerve monitoring may also be performed.

The fundamentals of this procedure are very similar to microvascular decompression for trigeminal neuralgia. Patients are positioned either semilateral or lateral, with the head in Mayfield pins turned to expose the retroauricular region. The head is usually tilted downward in order to improve the surgical angle to the lower cranial nerves. The ipsilateral shoulder is frequently taped down to improve the angle of visualization. The incision used may be either "C" shaped, linear, or "S" shaped, but it should always span the asterion so that the angle of the transverse sinus and sigmoid sinus can be defined in the bony opening. This angle must be developed to allow the surgeon access to the cerebellopontine angle, and although there is no need to reach the upper portion of the cistern, the exposure for a glossopharyngeal nerve operation is not fundamentally different from its trigeminal counterpart. Once the scalp is opened, the surgeon can perform either a craniotomy or a craniectomy, based on the sinus angle. The edges of the transverse and sigmoid sinuses should be seen after the bony removal is complete. The size of the cranial opening is variable, but it is usually around 3 cm in diameter. The mastoid air cells should be waxed. The dura is opened and CSF is allowed to drain, until which point the cerebellum relaxes and CSF spontaneously drains from the opening. At this point, the surgeon gently retracts the lateral portion of the lateral cerebellar hemisphere, proceeding under high magnification along the petrous face, until the facial and vestibulocochlear nerve complex comes into view. Just caudal to this nerve complex the surgeon will find the lower cranial nerves. The most rostral of these nerves will be the glossopharyngeal nerve, which runs as a single nerve bundle. The vagus nerve runs as several separate nerve rootlets into the same foramen just caudal to the glossopharyngeal nerve, as does the spinal accessory nerve. The glossopharyngeal nerve may be distinguished from the vagus by its single root, as well as by a slightly grayer color than the vagus. Once the nerves are identified, the surgeon may explore the root entry zone of the glossopharyngeal nerve, addressing any compressive etiologies along the way. Alternatively, the surgeon may coagulate and sharply divide the glossopharyngeal nerve. Typically, if a nerve section is performed, the surgeon will then also divide the upper 1/3 of the rootlets of the vagus nerve as well, since this portion of the vagus contains nerve fibers functionally identical to the glossopharyngeal nerve.

Following the completion of the decompression or the nerve section, the dura is closed. The bone flap may be replaced or a bone substitute used, but this is not a necessity. The incision is closed tightly in layers to reduce the risk of CSF leak.

Oral Boards Review—Management Pearls

1. Positioning of the head with adequate turning to expose the retroauricular region, and a downward tilt of the head to improve the surgical angle, are important.
2. BAER monitoring is useful to reduce the risk of hearing loss with surgery, as cerebellar retraction may cause unrecognized stretching of the nearby cochlear fibers.
3. The glossopharyngeal nerve appears as a single bundle, and is slightly greyer than the adjacent vagus nerve, which runs as multiple rootlets into the jugular foramen.
4. If a glossopharyngeal nerve section is performed, it is important to section the upper 1/3 of the nerve fibers of the vagus as well.

Pivot Points

1. If a patient presents with classic features of glossopharyngeal neuralgia, they should be considered early for either a MVD or intracranial glossopharyngeal nerve section.
2. Imaging may point to a vascular compression etiology for the neuralgia, but the decision to perform a MVD (rather than a nerve section) should take into account other factors, such as patient age and comorbidities.
3. BAER monitoring during surgery is an important safeguard against excessive retraction.

Aftercare

Patients are usually observed in an intensive care unit setting on the first night after surgery. They are mobilized as soon as possible and are usually allowed to leave the hospital in short order. A short course of steroids is often prescribed to lessen the incidence of aseptic meningitis after surgery. Routine imaging is not necessary. Small pseudomeningoceles are not uncommon, and they usually resolve spontaneously. It is uncommon to see any difficulties with swallowing even after glossopharyngeal nerve section, and when they do occur, they are typically self-limited.

Complications and Management

The most frequent complication of MVD surgery is aseptic meningitis, probably related to blood in the CSF or the presence of Teflon. Symptoms consist of headache, neck stiffness, and low-grade fever. The usual treatment of these symptoms consists of a short burst of steroids. Of course, on the differential for such symptoms is septic meningitis. If the patient presents with such symptoms but appears more ill than expected, or does not respond to steroids, a lumbar puncture is indicated to rule out infection.

Either microvascular decompression or glossopharyngeal nerve section may also be complicated by CSF rhinorrhea, usually related to CSF egress from the dural opening through a mastoid air cell into the middle ear and through the Eustachian tubes into the nasopharynx. When present, CSF rhinorrhea is relatively straightforward to manage, given the superficial nature of the CSF egress pathway. A lumbar drain may be placed temporarily to allow the hole in the mastoid air cell to seal, but if this does not resolve the issue, a superficial re-exploration, with resealing of the air cells will stop the leak.

Less frequent complications include hearing loss, facial paralysis, swallowing difficulties, hoarseness, or cerebellar infarction. Hearing loss may occur, especially in older patients. BAER monitoring is helpful to reduce the risk of this complication. If waveforms diminish during the surgical approach, it is advisable to temporarily cease manipulation and retraction and allow waveforms to recover before continuing. Facial paralysis is very unusual, and it is usually a sign of excessive retraction. It is frequently accompanied by significant hearing loss. Swallowing problems or hoarseness are distinctly uncommon, even if a nerve section is performed. Cerebellar stroke is usually a sign of significant cerebellar retraction, or suboptimal positioning at the start of surgery.

Oral Boards Review—Complications Pearls

1. Careful patient positioning is essential to improve visualization and reduce the need for cerebellar retraction during surgery, reducing the risk of the most serious complications of the operation.
2. The most common complications of MVD surgery, aseptic meningitis and CSF rhinorrhea, are relatively straightforward to manage.
3. BAER monitoring allows the surgeon to reduce tension on the facial and cochlear nerves, reducing the risk of cranial neuropathies as a result of surgery.
4. Lower cranial nerve dysfunction is uncommon, even if glossopharyngeal nerve section is performed. It is usually self-limited when it does occur.

Evidence and Outcomes

There are numerous small, retrospective series documenting a favorable success rate with either MVD or glossopharyngeal nerve section. While MVD of the glossopharyngeal nerve is attributed to Jannetta in 1977, the sectioning of the nerve intradurally was first proposed much earlier. In 1927, Walter Dandy proposed sectioning the glossopharyngeal nerve (along with the rostral fibers of the vagus). This operation has been in the neurosurgical armamentarium for decades, with pain relief usually over 90%. Recently, there has been interest in a more minimal sectioning procedure of the glossopharyngeal nerve alone, with the authors contending that the success rates rivaled the traditional combined nerve section, with a lower incidence of pharyngeal discomfort or dysphagia in the more limited procedure. MVD of the glossopharyngeal nerve has been reported in a number of small series, with success rates better than 90%, although the rate of lower cranial nerve deficit has been widely variable (as low as 0% and as high as 10%).

There also has been recent interest in gamma knife surgery, although the literature documenting results of this procedure is still too scant to effectively compare this procedure to the open procedures.

Further Reading

Dandy WE. Glossopharyngeal neuralgia (tic doloureaux). Its diagnosis and treatment. Arch Surg. 1927;**15**:198–214.

Laha RK, Jannetta PJ. Glossopharyngeal neuralgia. J Neurosurg. 1977;47:316–320.

Chen J, Sindou M. Vago-glossopharyngeal neuralgia: A literature review of neurosurgical experience. Acta Neurochir (Wien). 2015;157:311–321.

Héroux, F., & Mathieu, D. Treatment of glossopharyngeal neuralgia by gamma knife radiosurgery. *Can J Neurol Sci.; Le Journal Canadien Des Sciences Neurologiques.* 2015;*42*(5):350–352. http://doi.org/10.1017/cjn.2015.58

Trigeminal Neuropathic Pain

Mandana A. Behbahani, Nauman S. Chaudhry, and Konstantin V. Slavin

5

Case Presentation

A 62-year-old woman was referred for neurosurgical treatment of medically refractory pain in the right side of her forehead following a traumatic facial injury. The pain started almost immediately after a blunt injury of the right supraorbital region 4 years prior. The pain was described as constant, dull, and burning without any shooting attacks or focal triggers. Based on the patient's records, there was documented partial sensory loss in the area of pain for the first year after the injury; however, at the time of examination, her sensation was normal and symmetric to light touch, pinprick, and temperature, except for mild hyperesthesia and allodynia. There were no skin discolorations or trophic changes. The patient did not report any rash prior to development of pain or since the pain started.

Questions

1. What is the likely diagnosis?
2. What nerve/branch is likely to be involved in pain genesis?
3. What other conditions may be presenting with a similar clinical picture?

Assessment and Planning

Based on the patient's symptoms, one could arrive to the correct diagnostic impression of trigeminal neuropathic pain. Although the majority of facial pain patients that present to a neurosurgical practice may be labeled with a diagnosis of "trigeminal neuralgia," the clinical features and history should guide the examiner to properly classify the pain according to the widely accepted Burchiel facial pain classification (1). Generally, classical trigeminal neuralgia (TN) is characterized by spontaneous onset (Type 1 TN if the pain is predominantly episodic vs. Type 2 TN if the pain is predominantly constant) of attacks typically described as sharp, shooting or electric, in the distribution of one or several trigeminal nerve branches. *Trigeminal neuropathic pain* (TNP) and *trigeminal deafferentation pain* (TDP) develop after an injury to the trigeminal nerve itself. If the injury is unintentional, as it was in the case example above, then the pain is classified as TNP. If the nerve injury was an intentional part of surgical intervention to treat TN or other pain conditions, then the pain is classified as TDP. Other considerations may include *postherpetic neuralgia* (PHN), which occurs after an outbreak of shingles (herpes zoster), or *symptomatic* TN, a form of trigeminal neuralgia that occurs in the setting of an inciting illness such as multiple sclerosis. A separate category in the Burchiel classification includes *atypical facial pain*, when the location of pain does not match anatomic distribution of a specific nerve and the pain itself is related to an underlying somatoform pain disorder.

Oral Boards Review—Diagnostic Pearls

1. Diagnostic impression in facial pain should be based on pain description, history, and examination, followed by diagnostic imaging. A standard diagnostic algorithm would help in assigning the proper diagnostic category (2).
2. Presence of sharp, shooting episodes (electric-shock like attacks) strongly suggests diagnosis of TN. Idiopathic TN is further divided into types 1 and 2 based on predominance episodic and constant pain, respectively. Other entities known as symptomatic TN are seen in cases of multiple sclerosis (and other conditions such as cerebellopontine angle tumors, infections, and vascular and inflammatory processes, etc.) constitute a separate facial category.
3. Although TN is an excellent example of neuropathic condition, the term *trigeminal neuropathic pain* (TNP) is reserved for non-TN patients with known traumatic or unintentional surgical injury of trigeminal nerve or its branches. Typical descriptors of pain (constant, dull, burning, stinging) in combination with normal sensory examination, any degree of sensory impairment (from mild hypoesthesia to complete anesthesia), or additional sensory phenomena (hyperpathia, hyperesthesia, allodynia) are exactly the same for TNP, TDP, and PHN, but the difference is in the etiology of the condition (see previous discussion).
4. The involvement of a particular trigeminal branch in the pain generation/processing may be confirmed with a local anesthetic block, but the use of blocks is not mandatory for making the diagnosis.

The diagnosis and subsequent treatment may be determined with the aid of an established algorithm for the treatment of facial pain that includes a set of simple questions and decisions (2).

Once the diagnosis is established, the treatment options are considered based on the patient's overall medical condition, pain severity, and ability and willingness to undergo surgical intervention(s). Psychological testing is usually performed in order to assess the presence and extent of a patient's somatization, depression, cognitive impairment, etc. Prior to considering surgery for pain, one should try non-surgical treatments, including analgesic medications aimed at the treatment of neuropathic pain (anti-inflammatory, anticonvulsants, and antidepressants). In some cases, a corrective intervention that would eliminate the source of the nerve irritation may also be considered. In cases of TNP, a corrective surgery is rarely an option; usually, neurosurgical involvement starts after corrective surgery and medical treatment have already been tried and failed.

In this illustrated case, surgical intervention for pain relief should be seriously considered due to the disabling nature of the patient's pain, refractory medical treatment, lack of spontaneous improvement, and clear anatomical location of pain concordant with the distribution of the injured supraorbital nerve.

Questions

1. Is response to a nerve block predictive of success in neuromodulation procedure?
2. Would chronic pain stemming from injury of supraorbital nerve be considered an indication for surgery?
3. Would standard approach to surgical management of trigeminal neuralgia be appropriate in treatment of trigeminal neuropathic pain?

Decision Making

Surgical management of facial pain has been a subject of interest and fascination for neurosurgical community since the dawn of neurosurgery (3). Multiple treatment approaches have been developed to treat medically refractory cases of facial pain, including ablation, decompression, electrical modulation, and focused radiation aimed at the trigeminal nerve, its peripheral branches, the ganglion, and the nerve root. However, most of these surgical interventions were developed for the treatment of TN rather than other causes of facial pain, such as TNP.

Surgical options for TNP patients, similar to neuropathic pain syndromes in other parts of the body, include destruction and neuromodulation approaches. Although destructive procedures (neurotomy, neurectomy, ganglionectomy, and rhizotomy) have relatively limited value in the surgical management of TNP, electrical stimulation of trigeminal nerve is an accepted way to treat neuropathic pain in cases of TNP, TDP, and PHN. Since one may expect to achieve pain relief from stimulation at different points along the trigeminal system of nociception and pain processing, the decision making related to the exact stimulation target is guided by individual circumstances and feasibility. Stimulation of peripheral trigeminal nerve branches is expected to work when the patient has at least partial preservation of sensory function and when the branch to be stimulated is accessible and relatively immobile. Supraorbital and infraorbital nerves are considered excellent stimulation targets for supraorbital and infraorbital TNP, respectively, unless the patient has complete sensory loss in the area of pain.

In cases of complete numbness, the peripheral neuromodulation procedures (stimulation of trigeminal nerve/branches and ganglion) are more likely to fail, and therefore the surgical target choice becomes limited to motor cortex, sensory thalamus, or the uppermost cervical spinal cord, where the trigeminal nucleus caudalis is located. In cases of multiple branch involvement, trigeminal peripheral nerve stimulation (PNS) may become problematic due to a need in multiple electrodes placed over different branches. Gasserian ganglion stimulation may therefore be a preferred modality.

Currently, it is recommended to document pain improvement with a week-long stimulation trial using a temporary electrode before permanent implantation of a trigeminal PNS system.

Questions

1. Is trigeminal PNS considered a treatment option for medically refractory trigeminal neuralgia?
2. Would history of herpetic eruption rule out the possibility of improvement with trigeminal PNS?
3. Is there an established threshold in duration of pain to make patients more or less favorable candidates for neuromodulation?

Surgical Procedure

Implantation of a supraorbital PNS system may be done under sedation or under general anesthesia. Performing the procedure under sedation allows the surgeon to perform intraoperative testing, but patient cooperation may prove difficult in such settings. Performing the procedure under general anesthetic is better tolerated but requires radiographic confirmation of lead position spanning the supraorbital notch.

In preparation for surgery, the patient is positioned in such a way that the entire intended path of the stimulation system is within the sterile field and is easily accessible for surgical manipulation. With the intention of placing the implantable pulse generator (IPG) in the standard infraclavicular position, it is recommended to anchor the supraorbital PNS electrode in the retroauricular region. The retroauricular region serves two important purposes: (1) it provides for a relatively immobile area where there is a strong fascial layer to attach the anchors, and 2) it provides an easy trajectory for tunneling toward both the periorbital stimulation target and the infraclavicular IPG site. In the supine position, the patient's head is rotated toward the contralateral shoulder, and a roll is placed under ipsilateral shoulder to facilitate the electrode tunneling. There should be adequate room for the C-arm fluoroscopy device to be positioned around the patient's head to obtain an anteroposterior view of the skull.

The entry point for the electrode is chosen 1.5–2 cm lateral to the eyebrow, and once a small incision is made with a #15 blade, the needle from the electrode kit is inserted into the epifascial plane toward the midline and parallel to the superior edge of the orbit.

Oral Boards Review—Surgical Pearls

1. The needle from the electrode kit should be bent to create a curved trajectory for electrode insertion that conforms to the forehead curvature (Figures 5.1 and 5.2). After the needle is bent, the surgeon has to confirm that the stylet may be easily removed through the needle.
2. As opposed to the insertion of percutaneous spinal cord stimulation electrodes, where the epidural needle serves as an access tool and the final electrode placement is performed through fluoroscopically guided navigation of the wire-like electrode in the epidural space, in PNS the needle serves as the delivery tool, since the electrode cannot be advanced in the epifascial plane. Therefore, the needle tip should be positioned at the farthest end of the intended electrode trajectory (Figure 5.3). With this, it may be prudent to

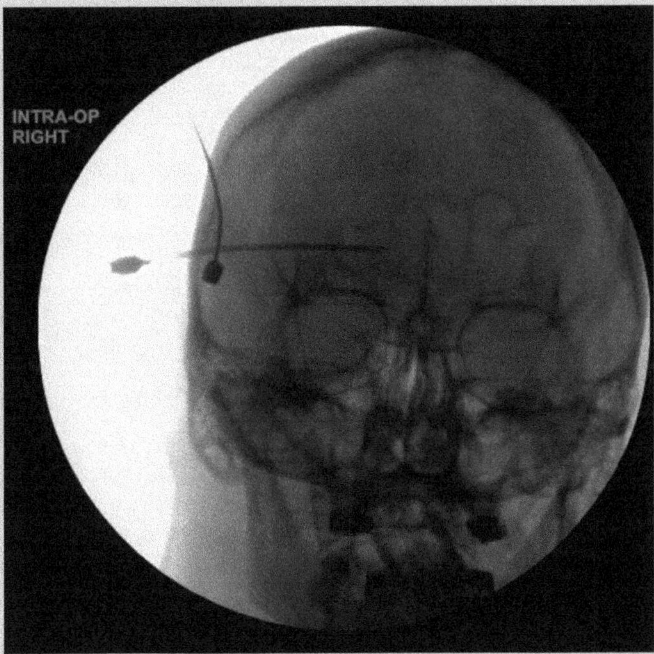

Figure 5.1. Intraoperative fluoroscopic image of the curved needle inserted over the projection of the right supraorbital nerve.

measure the distance of the subcutaneous (epifascial) path and make sure that the needle length and curvature would allow reaching the intended target from the skin incision.

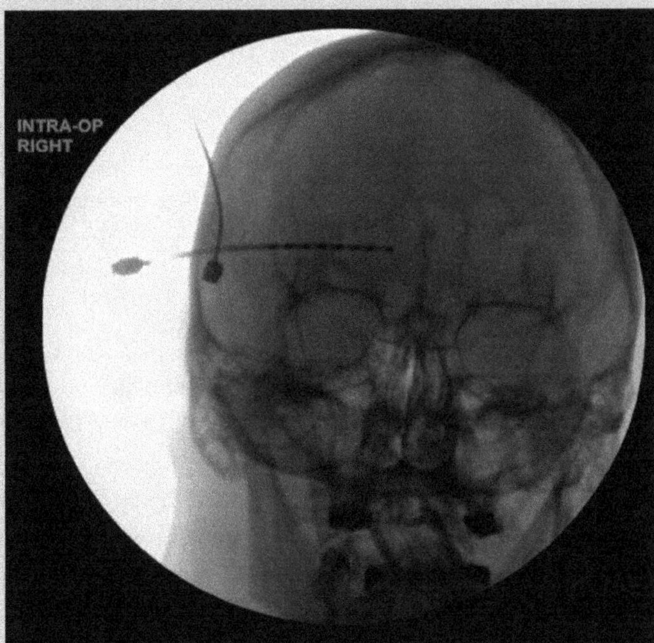

Figure 5.2. Intraoperative fluoroscopic image of the octopolar electrode within the insertion needle.

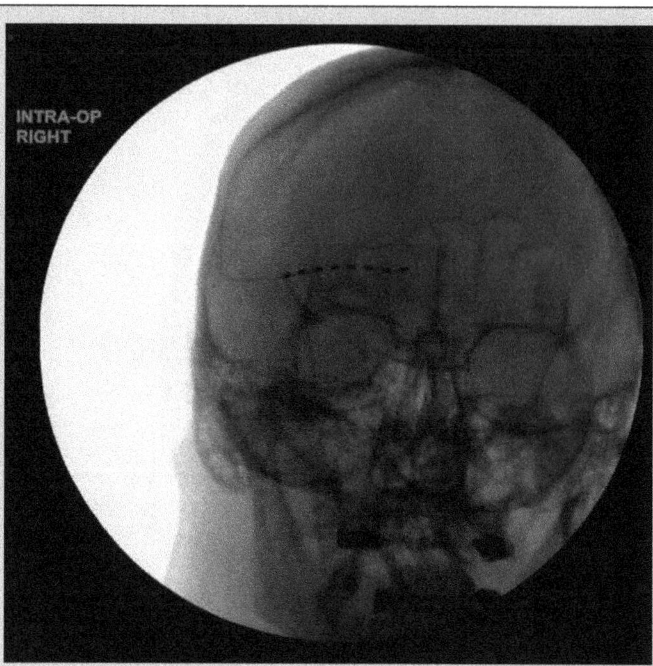

Figure 5.3. Intraoperative fluoroscopic image of the final position of the supraorbital nerve stimulation electrode.

3. For the same reason, the bevel of the curved needle should be facing away from the skin surface so the electrode does not create undue pressure on the skin upon leaving the needle.
4. The choice of the electrode is dictated by individual anatomy and pain pattern. Four-contact electrode may be sufficient for the unilateral stimulation, and 8- and 12-contact electrodes may be used for unilateral and bilateral coverage.

Once the electrode is positioned and its location is confirmed with fluoroscopy, the electrode tail is tunneled to the larger vertical incision behind the ipsilateral ear. The tunneling path goes above the ear, connecting the retroauricular and frontotemporal incisions. In the retroauricular incision, the electrode is anchored to the thick fascial layer and a strain-relief loop is created to reduce the risk of electrode migration. Non-absorbable synthetic braided polyfilament sutures are used to hold the anchor to the fascia. After anchoring, the electrode tail is passed through a dedicated tunneling tool to the infraclavicular IPG pocket. Throughout the anchoring and tunneling process, intraoperative fluoroscopy is used to confirm that the electrode contacts remain in the desired position overlaying the course of the supraorbital nerve.

Electrode connection to the IPG is tested with telemetry, and then, once the connection is secured with a locking screw, the excess of electrode is coiled under the generator and then the generator is secured to the underlying pectoral fascia using non-absorbable sutures. Once hemostasis is achieved and the incisions are irrigated with antibiotic solutions, the closure is done in standard layer-by-layer fashion.

The technique and process for insertion of the temporary (trial) and permanent electrodes is similar, with only a few small differences. For the trial electrodes, there is no need for distant tunneling, as the generator for the trial system is external. The temporary electrodes may be taped to the skin next to the entry point, or they may be tunneled away from the path of permanent implantation and sutured to the skin to minimize the possibilities of migration, pull-out, and infection.

Pivot Points

1. The trial success is determined by the degree of pain relief and absence of stimulation-related side effects. The usual cut-off for efficacy is greater than 50% reduction in pain intensity.
2. There is no consensus on whether patient-reported >50% improvement in pain intensity is a better indicator for success compared to >50% reduction in pain scale readings (Visual Analog Scale or Numeric Rating Scale) as there is a concern that pain severity in most scales does not follow a linear pattern. It is not uncommon for chronic pain patients to describe pain reduction from 9/10 to 6/10 on NRS while mentioning a 60 to 70% improvement in pain.
3. The lack of paresthesia in the area of pain may be expected to produce inadequate pain relief. The question in such a situation is whether lack of paresthesia is related to baseline impairment of sensation and inability of PNS to produce paresthesia or if the electrode position is suboptimal and has to be changed.
4. It is imperative to have the stimulation programming performed by qualified personnel. It is most valuable if the implanting surgeon performs or directly supervises PNS programming, as detailed knowledge of anatomy and spatial relationship between the electrode contacts and the targeted nerve(s) may be crucial in finding optimal stimulation settings.

Aftercare

The follow-up in TNP patients with implanted neurostimulators, including supraorbital PNS, includes reprogramming of the PNS system as needed for optimal coverage and pain relief, as well as occasional troubleshooting when the stimulation benefits fade or disappear. If the pain relief is sustained, then no particular follow-up is needed. The use of non-rechargeable IPG devices requires replacement on a regular basis, usually every several years. Of note, rechargeable IPGs also have a finite life; despite regular on-time recharges, most devices are expected to require replacement 6 to 10 years after original implantation.

Reprogramming is needed whenever the patient describes a change in paresthesia coverage—usually due to inevitable micro-migration of the electrode leads—and whenever the stimulation benefits wane despite adequate paresthesia, probably due to development of tolerance. The usual reprogramming includes changes in the stimulation parameters (frequency, pulse width, amplitude settings, polarity of the electrode contacts, cycling mode settings) and creation of different programs that the patients can choose from based on the pattern and severity of their pain.

It is not uncommon for TNP patients to experience gradual improvement of symptoms over time. In cases where patients have not been using PNS for more than 6 months because of the pain disappearance, the entire system may be safely removed.

Complications and Management

Most complications encountered with PNS in TNP patients have to do with the technical aspects of implantation and the device malfunction. In general, there may be hardware-related complications (e.g., device migration, fracture, disconnection, recharging issues), biological complications (e.g., erosion, infection, wound dehiscence, hematomas, seromas, pain, or discomfort around the device), and stimulation-related problems (e.g., muscle spasms, unpleasant paresthesias, and loss of pain relief).

As with any other surgical complications, it is worthwhile to place extra effort in prevention of complications rather than dealing with them after they occur. Proper anchoring and use of strain-relief loops are expected to reduce incidence of migrations and fractures. Eliminating excessive tension on the lead is likely to reduce incidence of disconnections.

The majority of stimulation-related issues may be corrected by reprogramming and changing the electrode polarity and other stimulation settings. If the stimulation-associated muscle spasms remain problematic despite reprogramming, then it may be prudent to consider repositioning the electrode into a more superficial tissue plane or in a higher part of the forehead away from the bulk of frontalis muscle.

Oral Boards Review—Complication Pearls

1. Although true infection of the implanted hardware must include device removal with possible re-implantation few weeks or months after the infection is resolved, more benign cases of suspected infection presenting with superficial redness and no drainage/fluctuance/purulence may be treated with a short course of systemic antibiotics and regular wound care.
2. The plane of insertion is the most important contributor to erosions and stimulation-related muscle spasms. Too superficial placement of a PNS electrode is expected to cause erosion over time, and too deep placement of the electrode under the fascia is likely to cause muscle spasms, particularly with high amplitudes that are required for stimulation to reach the sensory nerve.
3. Migrations may occur both as pull-outs and push-ins even with best anchoring techniques. Before proceeding with surgical revision, it is recommended to try to reprogram the device as sometimes benefits of stimulation may be recovered by changing the polarity of the contacts or widening the pulse width of stimulation. Cases of extreme migration may only be corrected with electrode repositioning.

Evidence and Outcomes

Although PNS for treatment of facial pain was first used in 1962 (4), there are no large-scale studies to evaluate its safety and/or efficacy for long-term TNP management. Most publications include a mixed patient population and concentrate on technical aspects of PNS rather than in-depth patient selection and predictors of success (5–10).

Published literature suggests that PNS works better for TNP than PHN (6) and that in patients with supraorbital TNP (referred to as "supraorbital neuralgia") pain relief is sustained for at least 6 months (9).

On a practical note, it is worth mentioning that supraorbital PNS is currently considered "off-label" for most neurostimulation devices. Recent introduction of dedicated, and FDA-approved, PNS devices may signal a change in the regulatory climate that changes how this therapy is labeled (11).

Further Reading

1. Burchiel KJ. A new classification for facial pain. Neurosurgery. 2003; 53:1164–1166; discussion 1166–1167.
2. Slavin KV, Nersesyan H, Colpan ME, Munawar N. Current algorithm for the surgical treatment of facial pain. Head Face Med. 2007; 3:30.
3. Eboli P, Stone JL, Aydin S, Slavin KV. Historical characterization of trigeminal neuralgia. Neurosurgery. 2009; 64:1183–1186; discussion 1186–1187.
4. Shelden CH, Pudenz RH, Doyle J. Electrical control of facial pain. Am J Surg. 1967; 114:209–212.
5. Dunteman E. Peripheral nerve stimulation for unremitting ophthalmic postherpetic neuralgia. Neuromodulation. 2002; 5:32–37.
6. Johnson MD, Burchiel KJ. Peripheral stimulation for treatment of trigeminal postherpetic neuralgia and trigeminal posttraumatic neuropathic pain: a pilot study. Neurosurgery. 2004; 55:135–141; discussion 141–142.
7. Slavin KV, Wess C. Trigeminal branch stimulation for intractable neuropathic pain: technical note. Neuromodulation. 2005; 8:7–13.
8. Slavin KV, Colpan ME, Munawar N, Wess C, Nersesyan H. Trigeminal and occipital peripheral nerve stimulation for craniofacial pain: a single-institution experience and review of the literature. Neurosurg Focus. 2006; 21(6):E5.
9. Amin S, Buvanendran A, Park KS, Kroin JS, Moric M. Peripheral nerve stimulator for the treatment of supraorbital neuralgia: a retrospective case series. Cephalalgia. 2008; 28:355–359.
10. Ellis JA, Mejia Munne JC, Winfree CJ. Trigeminal branch stimulation for the treatment of intractable craniofacial pain. J Neurosurg. 2015; 123:283–288.
11. Weiner RL, Garcia CM, Vanquathem N. A novel miniature, wireless neurostimulator in the management of chronic craniofacial pain: Preliminary results from a prospective pilot study. Scand J Pain. 2017; 17:350–354.

Postherpetic Neuralgia

Motor Cortex Stimulation and Nucleus Caudalis DREZ Lesioning

Sebastian Rubino, Roy S. Hwang, and Julie G. Pilitsis

6

Case Presentation

A 71-year-old male with a past medical history of right-sided medullary stroke, rheumatoid arthritis, coronary artery disease, left-sided acoustic neuroma resection, cutaneous T cell lymphoma, and a recent episode of a painful, right-sided facial rash presents with increasing facial pain. He describes the rash as erythematous, with groups of vesicles involving the right side of his forehead, brow, and extending down to the bridge of his nose, respecting the midline. Fortunately, he did not have any ocular involvement. He describes the painful sensation as deep aching and burning with episodes of numbness and tingling, painful to touch, exacerbated by light wind, pruritic at times, with electric shock-like pain that escalates upon repeated stimulation. The vesicles pustulated and crusted over after approximately 1 week, and the erythema also improved; however, the pain has persisted 3 months after the vesicles have healed and he reports the pain is worsening.

Questions

1. What is the differential diagnosis? Most likely diagnosis and why?
2. Did this patient exhibit Hutchinson's sign? Does this correlate with his presentation?
3. What is the most appropriate imaging modality to help guide treatment strategies?
4. What is the first line therapy for this diagnosis?

Assessment and Planning

The differential diagnosis for orofacial pain can be varied and includes classical and atypical trigeminal neuralgia, dental or boney pain secondary to dental pathology or osteomyelitis, short-lasting unilateral neuralgiform headache attacks with conjunctival injection and tearing (SUNCT) syndrome, short-lasting unilateral neuralgiform headache attacks with cranial autonomic symptoms (SUNA), cluster headaches, chronic paroxysmal hemicrania, giant cell arteritis, temporomandibular disorders, spread of the patient's cutaneous T cell lymphoma, multiple sclerosis, and postherpetic neuralgia (PHN) affecting the trigeminal nerve. While they all share some common symptomology, the differential can be heavily narrowed down based on the patient's history and physical exam; with attention devoted toward identifying the anatomical pain distribution, pain characteristics and course, dermatologic characteristics and course, age, and other systemic findings.

A functional way to characterize these diagnoses includes dividing them by those that have cutaneous manifestations versus those that do not and subsequently considering classic anatomical territories of involvement. Because many of these pain syndromes have various methods of presentation, patients often elicit the auspices of other physicians prior to ultimately being referred for neurosurgical evaluation. Therefore, it is prudent to obtain records and history of prior diagnostic work-up, as well as attempted therapies in order to most successfully establish the correct diagnosis.

Oral Boards Review—Diagnostic Pearls

1. The history and physical exam is the single most helpful tool in identifying the correct diagnosis, with the following definitions put forth by the Headache Classification Committee of the International Headache Society.[3]
   (a) **Classic Trigeminal Neuralgia**—includes at least three attacks of unilateral facial pain occurring in one or more divisions of the trigeminal nerve, with no radiation beyond the trigeminal distribution and pain having at least three of the following characteristics:
      i. recurrent paroxysmal attacks lasting from a fraction of a second to 2 minutes
      ii. severe intensity
      iii. electric shock-like, shooting, stabbing, or sharp in quality
      iv. precipitated by innocuous stimuli to the affected side of the face

      The distribution of pain usually occurs in the V2 and V3 divisions; does not cross midline; and rarely can occur bilaterally. There is usually a refractory period following a painful paroxysm, during which time the pain cannot be triggered.

   (b) **Painful Trigeminal Neuropathies**
      i. **PHN**—unilateral head and/or facial pain persisting or recurring for at least 3 months in the distribution of one or more branches of the trigeminal nerve, with variable sensory changes, and pain developing in temporal relation to acute herpes zoster infection. Typically occurs in the V1 distribution and is characterized by continuous deep aching, burning pain, paresthesias, dysthesias, hyperesthesias, electric shock-like pain, allodynia, pruritis, and wind-up pain. May also occur after an initial pain-free interval post-acute herpes zoster infection.
      ii. **Post-Traumatic**—unilateral facial or oral pain developing within 3 to 6 months following trauma to the trigeminal nerve
      iii. **Multiple Sclerosis**—characteristics of classical trigeminal neuralgia, induced by multiple sclerosis and associated with other signs and symptoms of multiple sclerosis

iv. **Space-Occupying Lesion**—characteristics of classical trigeminal neuralgia, induced by compression by a space-occupying lesion

(c) Headache Syndromes Involving V1 Distribution

i. Cluster headaches

ii. Short-lasting unilateral neuralgiform headache attacks with conjunctival injection and tearing (SUNCT)

iii. Short-lasting unilateral neuralgiform headache attacks with cranial autonomic symptoms (SUNA)

iv. Chronic paroxysmal hemicrania

v. Giant cell arteritis

(d) Other

i. T-cell Cutaneous Lymphomas—diverse entities with varied clinical presentations, one of which includes nodular or plaque-like lesions simulating panniculitis with most patients presenting with generalized lesions preferentially affecting the legs, arms, and trunk. Most patients present with systemic symptoms, lymphadenopathy, hepatosplenomegaly, cytopenias, and/or elevated liver function tests.[2]

ii. Dental Pathologies—more common in the V2 and V3 distributions

iii. Osteomyelitis—more common in the V2 and V3 distributions

2. PHN can develop after experiencing acute herpes zoster viral infection, which occurs with reactivation of the latent human herpesvirus 3 (same virus known to cause varicella) within dorsal root or trigeminal ganglia.
3. Hutchinson's sign is when there is involvement of the tip of the nose during acute herpes zoster ophthalmicus infection; thought to be a clinical predictor of ocular involvement.

MRI remains the best radiographic imaging modality to help rule out many of the diagnoses listed above. Trigeminal neuralgia is classically caused by vascular compression, multiple sclerosis plaque formation, and other lesional compression caused by tumors or infections, which can all be visualized by using appropriate MRI sequencing. The protocol used in our center includes a 3T MRI consisting of a thin section multiplanar steady-state free precession T2 weighted sequence, such as a fast imaging employing steady-state acquisition (FIESTA) sequence, through the brain stem to enhance contrast resolution between cerebrospinal fluid and the adjacent soft tissues, T1 weighted pre- and post-gadolinium sequences to evaluate for lesional enhancement, time-of-flight MR angiography, and a diffusion weighted image to evaluate for infarct. Protocols including the first 3 sequences have been shown to have 97% sensitivity and 50% specificity at detecting neurovascular compression.[4]

In the present case, all the MRI sequences, including the FIESTA sequence (Figure 6.1), were negative for any compressive, demyelinating, infectious, or infarction pathologies. Therefore, given this negative imaging and the patient's history of right-sided herpes zoster ophthalmicus, this patient most likely has PHN.

Medical management is the first-line therapy in both acute herpes zoster ophthalmicus and in subsequent PHN. Treatment with oral acyclovir within 3 days of acute zoster infection has been shown to shorten the duration of viral shedding, decrease

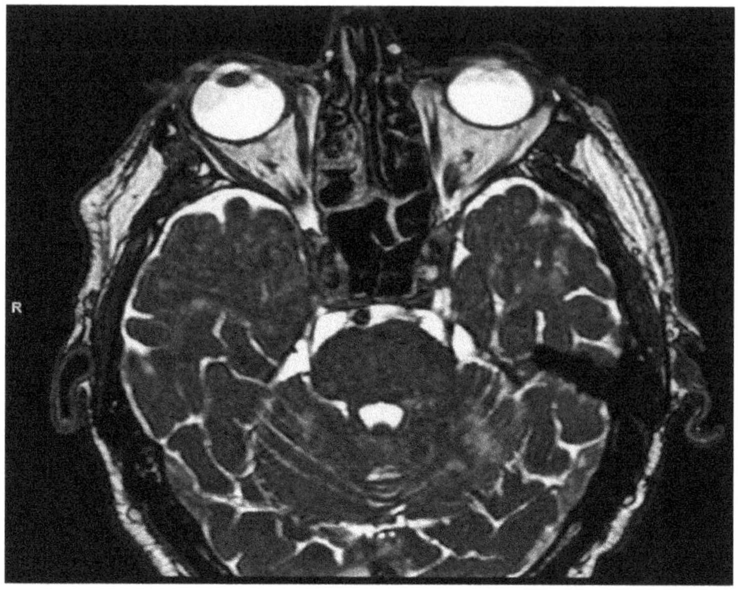

Figure 6.1. FIESTA MRI sequence negative for any compressive pathologies upon bilateral trigeminal nerves.

formation of new lesions, accelerate the rate of healing, and reduce the severity of acute pain.[5] However, there have been varied results regarding whether early treatment with antivirals also decreases the incidence of PHN. The zoster vaccine has been one of the only therapies proven to reduce overall incidence of herpes zoster by 51.3% and PHN by 66.5%.[6] Once a patient develops PHN, medical management includes gabapentin, pregabalin, tricyclic antidepressants, local anesthetics (topical lidocaine, capsaicin, piroxicam), and opioids.

Our patient was placed initially on gabapentin and then pregabalin, with no significant relief. He was unable to tolerate tricyclic antidepressants secondary to adverse side effects, including postural hypotension and confusion. Supplementation with topical, local anesthetics and opioids did not provide substantial pain relief.

Questions

1. What surgical interventions can be offered to patients with postherpetic trigeminal neuralgia who have failed medical management?
2. What is the proposed mechanisms of action of these interventions?

Decision Making

It is important to take a detailed history in order to correctly diagnose PHN and to avoid performing microvascular decompression, percutaneous trigeminal ganglion balloon compression, glycerol rhizolysis, or radiofrequency thermocoagulation procedures typically effective for classical trigeminal neuralgia and not PHN. Peripheral neurectomy, percutaneous gangliosis, sympathectomy, cordotomy, stereotactic trigeminal nucleotomy, peripheral nerve stimulation, nucleus caudalis dorsal root entry zone (NC

DREZ) lesioning, and motor cortex stimulation (MCS) have all been offered to patients suffering from PHN with varying degrees of success.

As reviewed by Kost and Strauss, acute herpes zoster infection leads to skin inflammation, denervation, peripheral nerve demyelination, Wallerian degeneration, and sclerosis; dorsal root ganglion inflammation, hemorrhagic necrosis, and neural loss; and spinal cord dorsal horn acute degeneration and unilateral segmental leptomeningitis with involvement of adjacent levels.[7] Postherpetic pain is the neuropathic pain that results from spontaneous peripheral neuron firing secondary to deafferentation, lower activation thresholds, and exaggerated responses all contributing to hyperexcitability of the dorsal horn. In NC DREZ lesioning, the goal is to target the secondary neuron, within the trigeminal thalamic pathway, upon which all these abnormal signals converge in order to limit aberrant hyperexcitability. Interestingly, the analgesic effect of MCS is less direct, and has been shown to activate horizontal interneurons that run parallel to the cortical surface and indirectly stimulate pyramidal tracts with generation of indirect waves at the spinal cord level; rather than directly stimulating pyramidal tracts.[8] These indirect networks of activation are the likely reason for increased regional cerebral blood flow in the ventrolateral and medial thalamus, insula, orbitofrontal cortex, cingulate gyrus, and upper brainstem during MCS,[9] and are likely to lead to modulation of secondary and tertiary neurons within the spinothalamic and trigeminal thalamic pathways.

Questions

1. In what anatomical location do you place the epidural paddle when conducting motor cortex stimulation for facial pain?
2. In what anatomical location do you make NC DREZ lesions?

Surgical Procedure

The pre-operative planning and intraoperative positioning, monitoring and procedural steps vary for motor cortex stimulator implantation and NC DREZ lesioning. Furthermore, post-operative programming is necessary to achieve optimal MCS.

Motor Cortex Stimulator Implantation

We perform motor cortex stimulator implantation using neuronavigation and intraoperative neuromonitoring with EMG testing and somatosensory-evoked potentials (SSEPs). The patient is initially positioned supine, with concomitant use of a contralateral shoulder bolster. The patient is fixed in place using a Mayfield 3-point fixation device, with his head turned toward the ipsilateral side of pain. Neuronavigation is registered and a preoperative plan localizing the hand-knob region is created. We identify the hand-knob motor region because of its known medial relationship to the facial motor region. Functional MR imaging is used to center our craniotomy over the hand region. The hand-knob is generally easier to visualize on MRI and appears omega-shaped on the precentral gyrus. Somatosensory evoked potential phase reversal is used intraoperatively to identify the precentral and post central gyrus. The facial motor region is then identified as lateral to the hand-knob region. We typically perform a 4 × 4 cm bone flap centered over the target, and place epidural tack-up sutures around the perimeter. We next place an electrode paddle over the hand knob region and look for SSEP signals showing phase reversal of the median nerve. We then place an electrode paddle with the same orientation and adjust the paddle slightly lateral so that the facial motor region corresponds to the center of the paddle. We place the paddle perpendicular to the motor strip along the inferior frontal sulcus. We then perform grid stimulation using monopolar stimulation until we elicit a facial EMG response. Our typical parameters are a frequency of 60 Hz, 300 ms pulse width, and voltage ranging from 1 to 5 V; beginning with a voltage of 1 and increasing in increments of 0.3 V. After obtaining the appropriate response, we then affix the paddle using 4-0 nylon sutures. We subsequently reaffix the bone flap using titanium plates. The wires exit the bone flap via one of the burr hole sites. We tunnel the wires toward the ipsilateral parietal area with serial relaxation loops placed, and proceed to place the impulse generator on the side ipsilateral to the facial pain.

Post-Operative Programming

There is a wide range of stimulation settings reported in the literature, with no clear stratification of what settings work best in different pathologies. Therefore, programming the stimulator can be quite challenging. Programming begins immediately post-operatively and often requires multiple programming sessions to achieve optimal pain control.

Nucleus Caudalis DREZ Procedure

We stabilize the patient using Mayfield 3-point fixation and place him in the prone position using chest rolls to decrease intrathoracic pressure. We mark the incision in the midline from the inion to the prominence of the C2 spinous process. We follow the nuchal fascia down the midline to the spinous process and perform subperiostial dissection to expose the spinous processes and laminae of C1 and C2, as well as the suboccipital area. Self-retaining retractors are placed and we proceed to perform a suboccipital craniotomy with C1 laminectomy. A durotomy is performed in a Y configuration and nylon sutures are used to fold back the dural folds. The circular sinus is clipped using hemoclips to prevent excessive bleeding. We are careful to preserve the subarachnoid plane as much as possible to prevent hemorrhage into the subarachnoid space and over-drainage of CSF until we are ready for DREZ lesioning. The two important landmarks to expose are the obex and the C2 rootlets. We use a 0.25 mm wide lesioning electrode and create 20 lesions, in 1 mm increments, in the interomediolateral sulcus from just above the obex to the level of the C2 rootlets. Each lesion is performed with the electrode tip set to 75° Celsius for 15 seconds. The probe is kept perpendicular to the medulla during the lesioning process. We use intraoperative neurophysiological monitoring of the cranial nerves and spinal cord. After the lesions are made, we copiously irrigate the surgical field, and subsequently perform a watertight dural closure using 5-0 Prolene suture. All additional tissue planes are reapproximated in layers.

Oral Boards Review—Operative Management Pearls

1. Functional MRI is critical for the identification of the hand-knob motor region and subsequent placement of the motor cortex stimulator paddle.
2. Correct localization of the facial region is marked by intraoperative stimulation, yielding an EMG motor response on the contralateral side.
3. The NC DREZ lesioning electrode must be inserted perpendicular to the medulla for best results.

Pivot Points

1. Post-operative programming remains challenging; there are no consistent programming settings. Patients must be pre-operatively counseled regarding the extended follow-up required for proper programming.
2. During programming, increases in stimulation settings may elicit seizures; therefore, programming should be performed in the presence of medical professionals.
3. NC DREZ lesioning is an invasive procedure that carries all the morbidities of posterior cervical surgery; therefore, it should be considered after all medical and other neurostimulatory therapies have failed. Careful preoperative assessment must be performed to limit morbidity and mortality.

Aftercare

For both procedures patients are admitted overnight for neurological monitoring. A fine-cut CT scan and x-rays of the stimulation system (Figure 6.2) are obtained post-operatively for patients undergoing MCS, while a standard cut CT scan is obtained post-operatively for patients undergoing NC DREZ. We also perform a postoperative non-contrasted cervical spine MRI, extending upward to the level of the rostral medulla, and including FLAIR, SWI, and DWI sequences. MCS patients are treated with prophylactic anti-epileptic medications for 7 days as per our routine for any craniotomy. NC DREZ patients require close monitoring of aspiration, given proximity to cranial nerves IX and X, for the first 2 to 3 days. We monitor patients closely until they are adequately tolerating food and liquids without dysphagia or aspiration.

Complications and Management

The most common complications of MCS vary, depending on the series, but include seizures, loss of effect, and stimulation site-induced pain. Seizures may occur during programming, so care should be taken to avoid motor effects, and programming should only be conducted in the presence of a health care professional. Other complications include epidural hematomas, equipment failure, and wound infections. Many of these complications can be mitigated using submotor threshold stimulation intensity and, if they occur, they typically can be resolved by decreasing stimulation intensity.

The most common complication of NC DREZ lesioning is mild to moderate transient ipsilateral limb ataxia, initially with rates as high as 90%, with groups

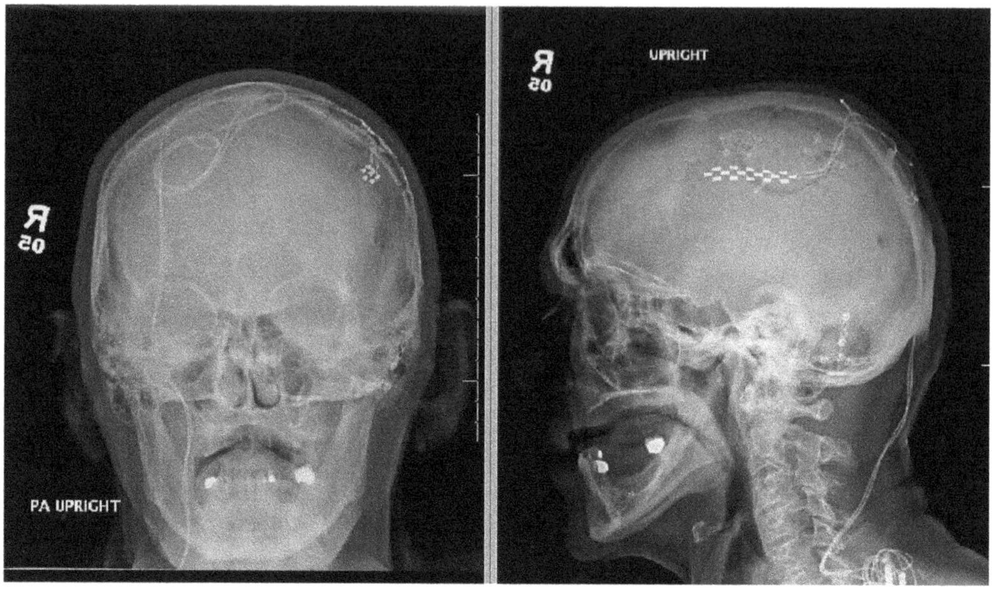

Figure 6.2. Post-operative skull x-rays showing final positioning of the MCS paddle.

reporting an occurrence rate as low as 18%.[10] This complication occurs due to involvement of ascending spinocerebellar fibers. If not present prior to surgery, this typically resolves within 1 month in 60% of patients, with some degree still being present at 1-year follow-up in 17% of patients.[11] Less commonly, transient ipsilateral hemiparesis may occur from edema involving the adjacent corticospinal tract. Cranial nerve dysfunction, corneal anesthesia leading to keratitis, and paralysis occur in less than 10%.[11]

It is important to counsel patients regarding post-operative facial sensation and success of pain relief. With success rates as high as 71% in patients with PHN,[12] it is important to note that hypo-algesia will be felt in all three trigeminal divisions. More favorable outcomes occur in patients with no sensory deficit or in those with involvement of only one trigeminal division. There have been single reports of patients experiencing intra-operative stroke, myocardial infarction, and death secondary to pulmonary embolism. These rare, severe complications may be mitigated with proper patient selection and optimization of pre-operative patient comorbidities.

Oral Board Review—Complications Pearls

1. Careful preoperative assessment and optimization will help minimize rare, severe complications described in the literature, including stroke, myocardial infarction, and pulmonary embolism.
2. MCS programming is often the time during which seizures occur. Therefore, care should be taken to avoid motor effects, and programming should only occur when a health care professional is present.
3. It is important to pre-operatively counsel patients regarding post-operative, self-limited ataxia and weakness after NC DREZ lesioning.

Evidence and Outcomes

W. Penfield and E. Boldrey were among the first to report sensory function of the motor cortex via direct stimulation of the precentral sulcus in 1937. While many animal and human studies since 1937 have furthered our understanding of pain physiology, T. Tsubokawa et al. were the first to introduce epidural motor cortical stimulation for the treatment of central deafferentation pain in 1991. Subsequently, B.A. Meyerson et al. were the first to report the efficacy of MCS for trigeminal neuropathic pain in 1993, with H. Ebel et al. reporting initial benefit in a patient with PHN. Given the low incidence of patients with facial, medication-refractory, PHN seeking neurosurgical care, there are no studies measuring outcomes solely in this patient population. The current literature consists of studies involving trigeminal neuropathic pain, within which several patients with PHN are included. In 2005, J.A. Brown and J.G. Pilitsis reviewed the literature and found 76% of their cohort, 29 of 38 patients, with neuropathic facial pain achieved greater than 50% pain relief from motor cortex stimulation; while in their series of 10 patients, 2 patients with PHN experienced 66–80% and 100% pain relief from MCS with mean follow-up at 10 months. In 2006, D. Rasche et al. performed MCS for trigeminal neuropathic pain (not specific to PHN) and found 50% of its cohort, 5 of 10 patients, to have greater than or equal to 50% pain reduction with mean follow-up of 3.6 years. A recent series published in 2018 by D. Henseen et al., showed that 70% of patients with central neuropathic pain had clinically relevant pain relief with mean Visual Analog Scale (VAS) score reduction of 54.5% at 3-year follow-up. These results were further substantiated in a literature review by D.C. Parravano et al., where patients with neuropathic CRPS, phantom limb, and facial pain had 75–90% reduction in VAS scores after MCS.

Tractotomy of the spinal trigeminal tract for treatment of trigeminal neuralgia was first described by O. Sjoqvist in 1938. In 1970, E.R. Hitchock and J.R. Schvarcz were among the first to report stereotaxic trigeminal tractotomy for the treatment of postherpetic facial pain; this involved making only 1 precisely placed lesion within the nucleus caudalis. M. Sindou and G. Fischer performed the first spinal DREZ lesion for cancer pain in 1972, and the procedure was further developed by B.S. Nashold et al. to include serial lesions within the intermediolateral sulcus by using a radiofrequency electrode in 1975. In 1984, the Nashold group subsequently applied this methodology to the trigeminal nucleus caudalis, making multiple lesions from C2 to obex. In 1995, J.P. Gorecki et al. reported 71% of patients with PHN had good or excellent pain relief at a mean of 3 months follow-up. Similarly, in 1997 J.R. Schvarcz reported 72% abolition of allodynia or marked reduction of background pain in patients with dysesthetic facial pain (26% of which had postherpetic pain) with a minimum of 4-year follow-up. In 2008, Y. Kanpolat et al. reported that patients with other chronic facial pain etiologies such as atypical trigeminal neuropathic pain, geniculate and glossopharyngeal neuralgia, and cancer pain had initial 72.5% pain-relief; with 62% still having relief at 1 year with NC DREZ lesioning. In 2015, S. Rahimpour and V. Patel reported 80% of their cohort, 4 of 5 patients, with atypical facial pain had significant pain relief at 3 months after endoscopic NC DREZ lesioning. In a detailed analysis of patient satisfaction, S. Chivukula et al. reported a mean 50% pain reduction in patients with PHN who underwent NC DREZ lesioning; with 1 patient (33%) having less than 1-year satisfactory pain relief,

1 patient (33%) having 1 to 5 years of satisfactory relief, and 1 patient (33%) receiving greater than 5 years relief. Interestingly, 100% of the patients were either satisfied or very satisfied with the outcomes and 66% said they would have the procedure again.

Conclusions

Patients with medication-refractory PHN may be candidates for neurosurgical interventions, including MCS and NC DREZ lesioning. Given the low incidence of patients with medication-refractory PHN presenting for neurosurgical evaluation, the data for both procedures in this very specific cohort of patients are limited, particularly with regards to long-term outcomes. Additional research, patient follow-up, and community outreach must be undertaken to better understand procedural efficacy and, subsequently, to better make these therapies available to those in need of them.

Further Reading

1. Alicino C, Trucchi C, Paganino C, et al. Incidence of herpes zoster and post-herpetic neuralgia in Italy: results from a 3-years population-based study. *Hum Vaccin Immunother.* 2017;13(2):399–404.
2. Willemze R, Jansen PM, Cerroni L, et al. Subcutaneous panniculitis-like T-cell lymphoma: definition, classification, and prognostic factors: an EORTC cutaneous lymphoma group study of 83 cases. *Blood.* 2008;111(2):838–845.
3. Headache Classification Committee of the International Headache S. The international classification of headache disorders, 3rd edition (beta version). *Cephalalgia.* 2013;33(9):629–808.
4. Brinzeu A, Drogba L, Sindou M. Reliability of MRI for predicting characteristics of neurovascular conflicts in trigeminal neuralgia: implications for surgical decision making. *J Neurosurg.* 2018:1–11.
5. Cohen JI. Herpes zoster. *N Engl J Med.* 2013;369(18):1766–1767.
6. Oxman MN, Levin MJ, Johnson GR, et al. A vaccine to prevent herpes zoster and postherpetic neuralgia in older adults. *N Engl J Med.* 2005;352(22):2271–2284.
7. Kost RG, Straus SE. Postherpetic neuralgia—pathogenesis, treatment, and prevention. *N Engl J Med.* 1996;335(1):32–42.
8. DosSantos MF, Ferreira N, Toback RL, Carvalho AC, DaSilva AF. Potential mechanisms supporting the value of motor cortex stimulation to treat chronic pain syndromes. *Front Neurosci.* 2016;10:18.
9. Garcia-Larrea L, Peyron R. Motor cortex stimulation for neuropathic pain: from phenomenology to mechanisms. *Neuroimage.* 2007;37 Suppl 1:S71–79.
10. Kanpolat Y, Tuna H, Bozkurt M, Elhan AH. Spinal and nucleus caudalis dorsal root entry zone operations for chronic pain. *Neurosurgery.* 2008;62(3 Suppl 1):235–242; discussion 242–234.
11. Bullard DE, Nashold BS, Jr. The caudalis DREZ for facial pain. *Stereotact Funct Neurosurg.* 1997;68(1–4 Pt 1):168–174.
12. Gorecki JP, Nashold BS. The Duke experience with the nucleus caudalis DREZ operation. *Acta Neurochir Suppl.* 1995;64:128–131.

Occipital Neuralgia

Richard L. Weiner

7

Case Presentation

A 54-year-old right-handed female presents with a 15-year history of progressive, bilateral occipital headaches without known etiology. These headaches have become weekly in frequency, lasting 3 to 4 days at a time. She describes sharp, electric shock sensations with certain head movements followed by throbbing pain. The pain extends from either side of the midline at approximately C1 level superiorly to the bi-parietal regions. She occasionally notes pain to the supraorbital regions bilaterally as well. She initially responded to Imitrex and was diagnosed as having migraine headaches by a neurologist. Topamax was added as a headache preventative but she became overmedicated with severe cognitive side effects and "rebound" headaches. A second neurologist weaned her off all medications and has been treating her with monthly bilateral occipital nerve local anesthetic and steroid injections, which improve her headaches for several weeks. Without injections or medications her pain scale rating is 8/10. With injections she notes her pain rating reduces to 1–2/10 with gradual pain recurrence over several weeks. The patient is seeking a surgical opinion/solution for her chronic, intractable, bilateral occipital pain.

Questions

1. What is the most likely diagnosis?
2. Differential diagnoses?
3. Are imaging studies appropriate for this condition?
4. Which studies would you order?

Assessment and Planning

The differential diagnosis of chronic headaches can be quite complex and even confusing to both the neurologist and neurosurgeon. This patient presents with specific site pain in the region of the greater occipital nerves bilaterally. She has responded well to monthly local anesthetic injections into the region of the greater occipital nerves, suggesting these nerves are definitely involved in her headache syndrome. This clinical history strongly suggests the diagnosis of bilateral occipital neuralgia.

Occipital neuralgia is a distinct type of headache characterized by piercing, throbbing, or electric-shock-like pain in the upper neck, back of the head, and behind the ears, more frequently unilateral but occasionally bilateral. Typically, the pain of occipital neuralgia begins in the neck and then spreads upward. Some individuals also experience pain in the scalp, forehead, and behind the eyes. Their scalp may also be tender to the touch, and their eyes especially sensitive to light. The location of pain is related to the areas supplied by the greater and lesser occipital nerves, which run from the area where the spinal column meets the neck, up to the scalp at the back of the head. The pain is caused by irritation or injury to the nerves, which can be the result of trauma to the back of the head, compression of the nerves by upper cervical muscle spasms, or osteoarthritis, tumors, infection, hemorrhage, systemic disease, or other types of lesion impingement in the region of C2-3. Localized inflammation or infection, gout, diabetes, blood vessel inflammation (vasculitis), and frequent lengthy periods of keeping the head in a downward and forward position are occasionally associated with occipital neuralgia. In many cases, however, no cause can be found. A positive response (relief from pain) after an anesthetic nerve block will confirm the diagnosis of occipital nerve involvement.

Oral Boards Review—Diagnostic Pearls

1. Pain is in the distribution of the greater, lesser, and/or third occipital nerves (greater occipital nerve involvement on one side is most common presentation).
2. Attacks are episodic and last a few seconds to minutes followed by a chronic painful sensation radiating superiorly above the low occipital region. Pain is piercing, stabbing, or sharp in quality, and severe in intensity. Unpleasant sensations in the region of the occipital nerves may occur. Severe tenderness may be felt over the affected nerves.
3. Paroxysmal pain (as in trigeminal neuralgia) is often considered classic occipital neuralgia, although it may also be a trigger for chronic headaches.
4. Cervical and brain MRI studies with and without contrast should be performed to evaluate possible etiologies other than nerve root irritation for chronic headaches.
5. All patients should undergo preoperative neuropsychological testing to prevent surgical intervention in the presence of severe depression or other significant psychological issues.
6. Obtain a careful medication history. Patients on chronic opioids do not do as well with any type of neurostimulation.

Decision Making

The neurosurgical literature has tended to diagnose localized occipital pain as occipital neuralgia. Occipital nerve neurolysis and/or neurectomy have been part of the neurosurgical armamentarium for treating intractable occipital headaches for many years. Though occasionally very effective, it may occasional result in the development of delayed deafferentation pain in the distribution of the affected occipital nerve. This limits the long-term usefulness of these destructive procedures. C2 ganglionectomy for posttraumatic C2 pain syndromes has resulted in an 80% good to excellent outcome with a 3-year follow-up (Acar et al., 2008). Patients with non-traumatic C2 pain do not fare nearly as well as those with traumatic C2 pain and subtle but significant morbidity, including postoperative dizziness or gait disturbances, may be a persistent problem. It is not a recommended procedure due to its destructive nature.

C2 nerve decompression achieves up to a 79% success rate with 33% pain complete pain relief and 46% adequate pain relief over 2 years (Choi et al., 2015). C1-2 fusion corrects focal instability and may be indicated on rare occasion. C1-3 posterior rhizotomy via ventrolateral dorsal root entry zone lesioning at C1-3 can be an effective but highly invasive surgical technique.

All these surgical procedures, however, are quite invasive with potentially serious and permanent side effects.

Neuromodulation

Neuromodulation for treatment of chronic pain disorders over the past 40 years has centered on spinal cord stimulation (SCS) and peripheral nerve stimulation (PNS) of specific nerves that use implanted electrode and generator devices to modulate perception of abnormal pain signals to the brain. PNS implants originally required exposure of the affected nerve with placement of either coiled or paddle electrodes adjacent to the site of injury or involvement. Picaza (1977) reported pain suppression by PNS on six patients with occipital neuralgia using a cuff electrode technique with 50% of patients reporting a good outcome. Waisbrod (1985) reported a very good result from stimulation of the greater occipital nerve for painful peripheral neuropathy. In 1999 Weiner and Reed reported the first successful neurostimulation and control of occipitally mediated, headache pain with a percutaneous electrode placement technique at or near the level of C1 in the vicinity of the greater and or lesser occipital nerves within the subcutaneous tissues. This occipital nerve stimulation (ONS) technique started a rebirth of interest in PNS implants as an effective and relatively simple treatment for a variety of peripheral nerve chronic pain syndromes in addition to occipital headaches.

The attractiveness of neurostimulation lies in the fact that the surgical procedure and stimulation are relatively straightforward and reversible.

Occipital Nerve Anatomy

The greater occipital nerve is the medial branch of the dorsal primary ramus of the C2 spinal nerve. This nerve arises between the first and second cervical vertebrae, along with the lesser occipital nerve. It passes through the semispinalis and trapezius musculature just inferior to the superior nuchal line, then continues superiorly above the fascia and below the galea with several branches innervating the skin along the posterior part of the scalp to the vertex and extending laterally to the ear. It is the superficially traversing occipital nerves above their emergence from the trapezius fascia at the occipital protuberance that are targeted with subcutaneously placed electrodes for neurostimulation. See figures 7.1, 7.2, 7.3 and 7.4.

Surgical Procedure

Surgical placement of ONS leads has been modified somewhat by various implanters since it was first introduced in 1999. All patients undergo a 5- to 7-day trial with

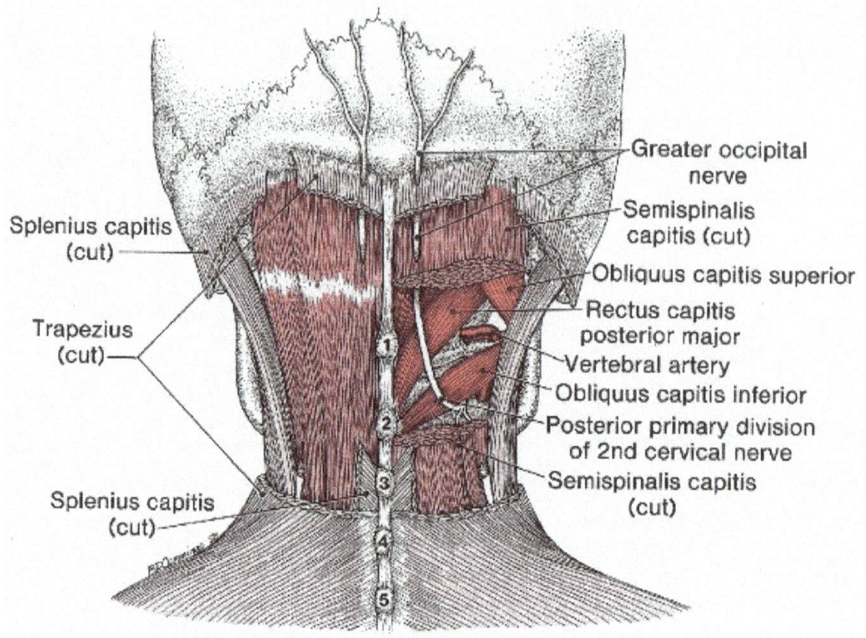

Figure 7.1. Anatomy of the greater occipital nerve.

externalized leads to assess ONS response. The trial lead placement is the same as described in the next section except the leads are fixed to the skin with anchors and secured for external cable connection. Trial leads can be placed via needle punctures rather than incisions. After removal of the trial leads, a 2-week waiting period should allow the superficial entry wounds to heal to minimize risks of subsequent infection.

The patient may be positioned laterally or prone, depending on the incision entry point and airway requirements. For patients undergoing unilateral occipital or frontal

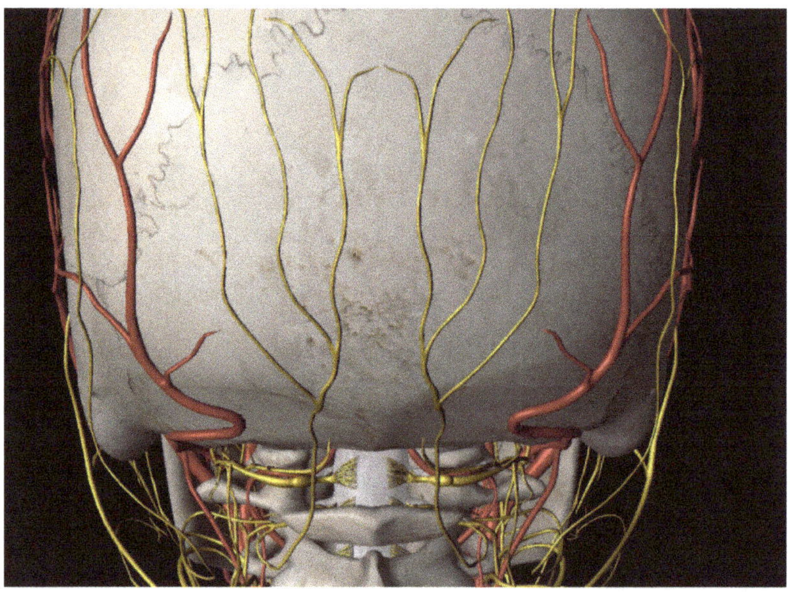

Figure 7.2. Schematic visualization of occipital nerve complex arising from C2.

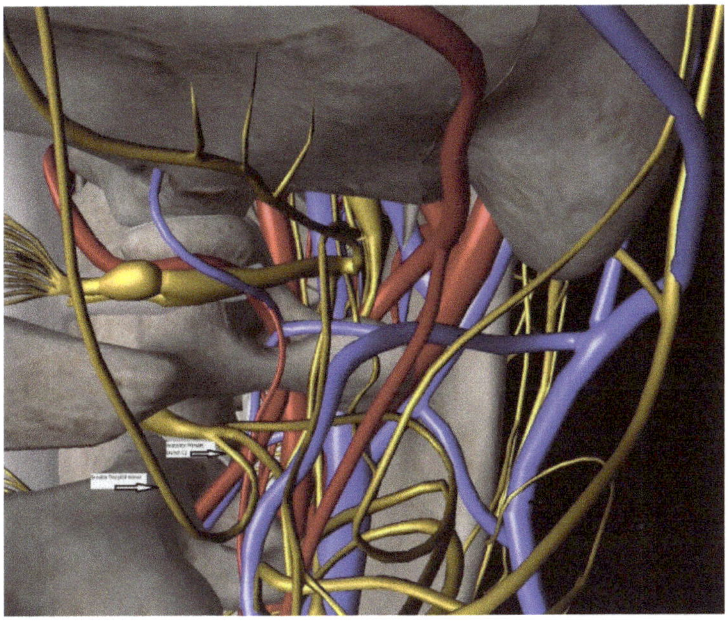

Figure 7.3. Close-up of GON origin at posterior rami of C2.

and occipital lead placement, a supine position with the head turned 90 degrees to the opposite side will facilitate placing the generator into the ipsilateral upper anterior chest region. Using local anesthesia at the incision site only, a vertical 2 cm incision is made at the level of the C1 lamina either medial and inferior to the mastoid process or in the midline posteriorly under fluoroscopic control, extending to, but not into

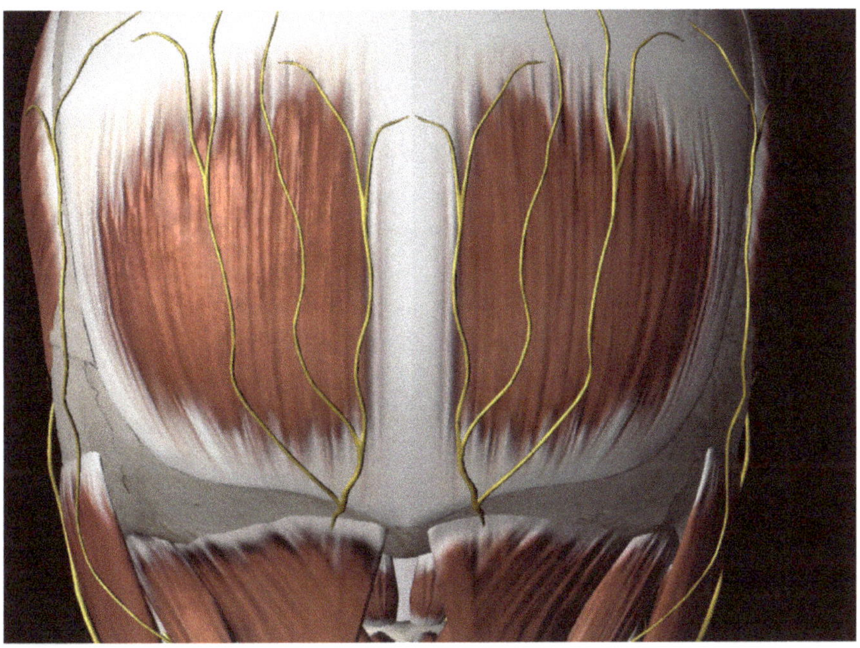

Figure 7.4. Occipital nerve complex superficial to the fascia at the inion and cephalad.

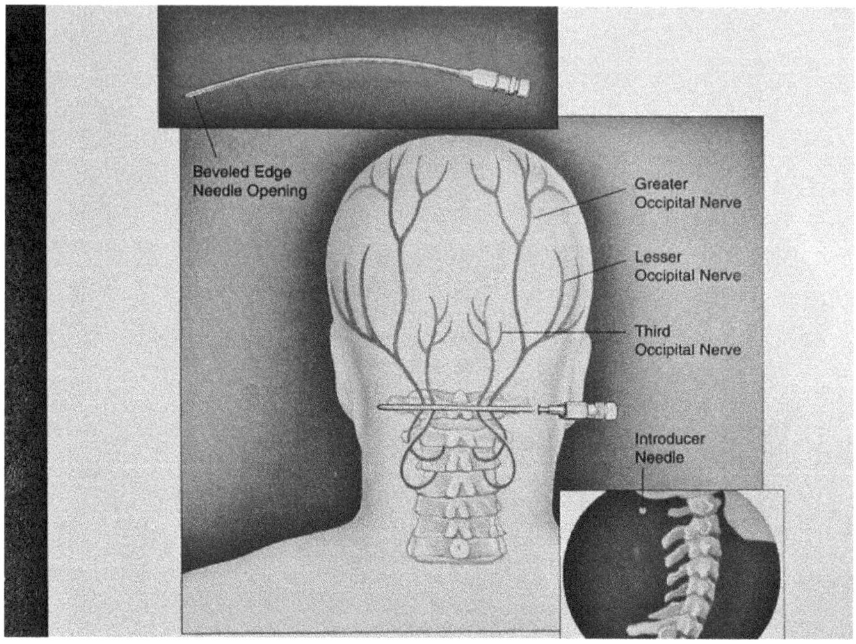

Figure 7.5. Curved needle placement for occipital nerve electrode coverage.

the cervicodorsal fascia. The subcutaneous tissues immediately bilateral to the incision are undermined sharply to accept a loop of electrode created after placement and tunneling to help prevent electrode migration. A Tuohy or Coude RX-2 (Epimed) needle is gently curved to conform to the transverse, posterior cervical curvature (bevel concave) and without further dissection is passed transversely in the subcutaneous space across the base of the affected greater and/or lesser occipital nerves, which at the level of C1 are located within the cervical musculature and overlying fascia. Single or dual 4- or 8-contact electrodes may be passed from the midline incision to either affected side or alternatively placed to traverse the entire cervical curvature bilaterally from a single side or via two opposing incisions. Surgical paddle electrodes can also be implanted subcutaneously, although somewhat more invasively, by using sharp dissection techniques with the electrode contacts oriented toward the fascia.

Rapid needle insertion, staying within the subcutaneous tissues, usually obviates the need for even a short-acting, general anesthetic once the surgeon becomes facile with the technique. Local anesthetic along the needle tract is not recommended so as to avoid tissue distortion and incomplete, on-the-table, stimulation response. Following placement of the electrode into the Tuohy or Coude needle, the needle is withdrawn and the electrode connected to an extension cable for intraoperative testing. See Figures 7.5, 7.6, 7.7, and 7.8.

Intra-Operative Stimulation Testing

After lead placement, stimulation is applied by using a temporary RF transmitter to various select electrode contact combinations that enable the patient to report, while awakened on the table, the stimulation location, intensity, and overall sensation (paresthesias). Most patients report an immediate stimulation in the selected occipital

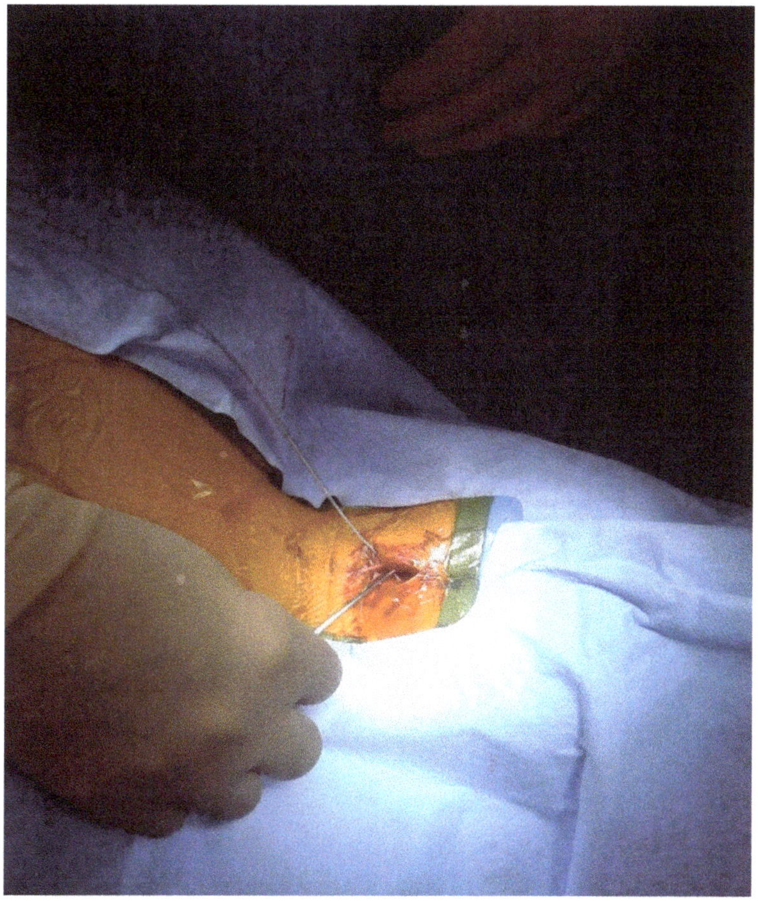

Figure 7.6. Second needle placement aimed at the contralateral mastoid area.

nerve distribution with voltage settings from 1 to 4 volts with midrange pulse widths and frequencies. A report of burning pain or muscle pulling should alert the surgeon the electrode is probably placed either too close to the fascia, intramuscularly, or too far above or below the C1 level and should be repositioned. Repeated needle passage for electrode placement can lead to subcutaneous edema and/or hematoma formation with loss of electrode conductivity, thereby blocking evaluation for permanent lead positioning.

Electrode Fixation and Tunneling

Probably the most important aspect of the procedure involves techniques to prevent electrode migration (pullback) from its transverse subcutaneous position in the highly mobile upper cervical region. Following successful stimulation, the electrode is sutured to the underlying fascia with the manufacturer-supplied, silicone fastener and 2-0 silk sutures. A small dab of medical grade, silicone glue can be placed between the anchor and electrode by using a small angiocath to ensure fixation. Some of the newer anchors on the market can be secured tightly to the electrodes with either an injection technique or small screws. A loop of electrode is also sutured in the previously prepared subcutaneous pocket to reduce migration risk as well. This allows for strain relief to mitigate

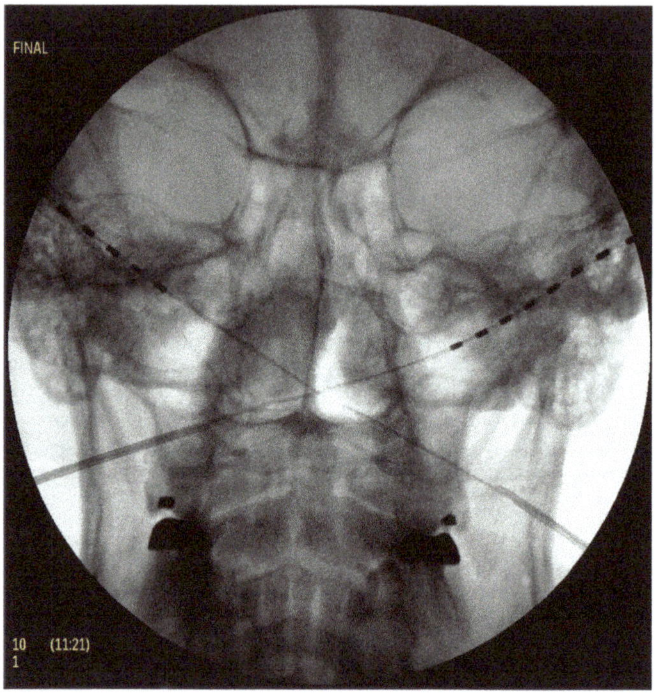

Figure 7.7. C1 entry point with angled subcutaneous tissue placements bilaterally.

the stress of cervical motion. A short-acting general anesthetic is used to tunnel the electrode(s) or extender wire to the distal site for connection and implantation of the receiver or generator.

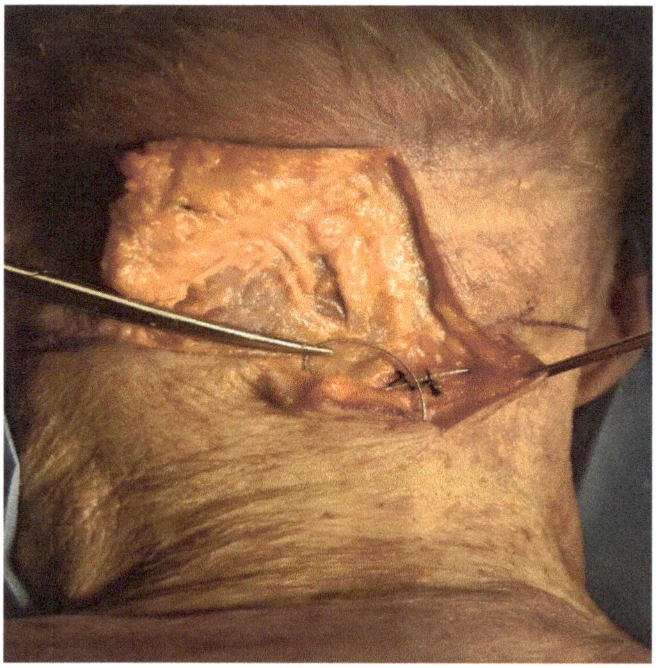

Figure 7.8. Secured anchor and leads into right-sided subcutaneous tissues. Left lead traversing occipital nerve complex.

Implantable Pulse Generator Implantation

There are three options available for the system power source: an external RF transmitter/receiver system, a primary cell implantable pulse generator (IPG), and a rechargeable IPG. The RF and rechargeable systems generally allow for more continuous, higher voltage outputs, while the primary cell requires less programming interaction. Most patients currently opt for the IPG system, which is currently an off-labeled application for peripheral use. With the voltage settings usually required for occipital stimulation, the primary cell lithium ion battery can last 3 to 5 years while the rechargeable may last 7 to 9 years before replacement.

Generator placement appears to influence both the patient's positioning during the procedure and the risk of postoperative migration, particularly if strain relief is not generously applied. Typical implant locations are

1. Upper buttock—facilitates single-stage electrode and generator placement in the prone position.
2. Abdomen—usually done with the patient in the lateral position.
3. Upper chest—lateral or supine positions favor this location.

There is significant, extension wire stretching with upper buttock generator placement when a patient bends forward that creates excessive tugging on the suboccipitally placed electrodes. This could be one of the major factors, along with anchoring technique, causing electrode migration. Thus, abdominal or anterior chest placement might reduce migration potential.

Summary of Technique Elements

- Signed consent including off label designator if applicable
- Prone, lateral, or supine positioning
- Map out occipital points of maximal tenderness with marker
- Short-acting sedation with airway preservation
- Local anesthetic to incision area. Avoid local to entire needle tract
- Curved Tuohy or Coude needle placement into subcutaneous tissues
- C1 starting point with midline or lateral incisions
- From midline, aim laterally or to mastoid processes bilaterally
- Advance needle subcutaneously, avoiding puncturing fascia or skin
- Needle should traverse several centimeters beyond mapped point so that the electrode can be pulled back during testing if coverage is incomplete
- Remove needles to uncover contacts and stimulate with patient awake
- Following optimal testing, fixate with loops and supplied anchors
- Create generator pocket: upper buttock, chest, or abdomen
- Tunnel extensions, connect, and close all wounds, dressings
- Maintain meticulous sterility throughout to minimize infection

Oral Boards Review—Management Pearls

1. Care must be taken to keep the Tuohy needle within the subcutaneous tissues. Muscle spasms will occur if an electrode is placed too deep within the muscle and erosion can occur if the electrodes are placed too superficially.
2. Strain-relief loops, along with secure anchor suturing, will reduce lead migration.
3. Be vigilant when tunneling in the occipitocervical region to avoid accidental intradural or even intracranial placement of the tunneling tip.
4. Maintain strict aseptic technique during the entire procedure, especially avoiding contamination of the IPG during implantation into the generator pocket.

Pivot Points

1. A 5- to 7-day trial of temporary occipital stimulation is necessary to assess patient suitability and pain response for permanent ONS placement.
2. Collaboration with a headache neurologist is beneficial throughout all aspects of patient selection and aftercare.
3. Neuropsychological testing is helpful to screen out inappropriate patient selection.

Aftercare

ONS implantation surgery is usually an outpatient procedure; however, mitigating circumstances could include excessive postoperative pain from surgical dissection for paddle placements and operating on patients with long-term narcotic intake and tolerance issues. These patients might require a more extended hospital stay for pain stabilization. Many implanters will use cervical collars for several weeks to help minimize excessive neck movements postoperatively. Patient instructions, including recharging procedures, should probably be reiterated either in person or over the phone a day or two after the procedure, as many patients have difficulty handling information following same day sedation. Dry, sterile dressing changes are important to minimize wound infection.

Complications and Management

Many reported studies on ONS include consequential adverse events. Complication rates of up to 33% have been reported in the literature with some revision rates approaching 60%. The most common complications include

- Infection
- Lead migration, breakage, erosion
- Persistent implant site discomfort
- Loss of effectiveness
- Frequent revisions

Most of these events are hardware or technique related and most likely from the application of SCS technology into a region of the body for which they have not been optimally designed. The posterior neck region can be highly mobile, producing significant strain on leads and extensions ultimately anchored at some distance away from the IPG. Infection seems to occur either at the generator site or adjacent to lead erosion. Seemingly normal skin flora, that is, Staphylococcus epidermidis, can become pathogenic, requiring meticulous care in manipulating the generator into place. Advances in hardware technology are beginning to address these issues including the development of wireless stimulation devices that do not require tunneling and placement of an IPG.

Oral Boards Review—Complications Pearls

1. Frequent complications include infection, electrode migration, electrode erosion, and generator site pain.
2. Each of these issues can be reduced in occurrence with meticulous surgical technique, attention to tissue planes, and avoidance of damage to the subdermal skin layers during needle placement.

Evidence and Outcomes

Outcome data from three multicenter, industry-sponsored studies have provided significant insights into the limitations of ONS implantation for a heterogeneous population of chronic headache patients.

The ONSTIM 2010 Study (Medtronic, Inc.)

Methods: A multicenter, blinded, randomized, controlled, (RCT) feasibility study was conducted to obtain preliminary safety and efficacy data on (ONS) for chronic migraine (CM) patients. Eligible subjects had greater than 15 days per month headaches and received an occipital nerve block. Responders to the blocks were randomized to adjustable stimulation (AS), preset stimulation (PS), or medical management (MM) groups.

Results: Seventy-five of 110 subjects were assigned to a treatment group; complete diary data were available for 66. A *responder* was defined as a subject who achieved a 50% or greater reduction in number of headache days per month or a three-point or greater reduction in average overall pain intensity when compared with baseline. Three-month responder rates were 39% for AS, 6% for PS, and 0% for MM. No unanticipated adverse device events occurred. Lead migration occurred in 12 of 51 (24%) subjects.

Conclusion: The results of this feasibility study offer promise and should prompt further controlled studies of ONS in CM.

St. Jude 2012

Methods: In this multicenter RCT, patients diagnosed with CM were implanted with a neurostimulation device near the occipital nerves and randomized 2:1 to active

(n = 105) or sham (n = 52) stimulation. The primary endpoint was a difference in the percentage of responders (defined as patients that achieved a ≥ 50% reduction in mean daily visual analog scale scores) in each group at 12 weeks.

Results: There was not a significant difference in the percentage of responders in the Active when compared with the Control group (95% lower confidence bound of −0.06; p = 0.55). However, there was a significant difference in the percentage of patients that achieved a 30% reduction (p = 0.01). Importantly, when compared with sham-treated patients, there were also significant differences in reduction of number of headache days (Active Group = 6.1, baseline = 22.4; Control Group = 3.0, baseline = 20.1; p = 0.008), migraine-related disability (p = 0.001), and direct reports of pain relief (p = 0.001). The most common adverse event was persistent implant site pain.

Conclusion: Although this study failed to meet its primary endpoint, this is the first large-scale study of PNS of the occipital nerves for CM patients that showed significant reductions in pain, headache days, and migraine-related disability. Additional controlled studies using endpoints that have recently been identified and accepted as clinically meaningful are warranted in this highly disabled patient population with a large unmet medical need.

A 1-year follow-up, safety, and efficacy study by the St. Jude study group is the first large-scale, prospective, controlled study evaluating PNS in the occipital region for CM. Several observations from the study are reported here for consideration:

- PNS in the occipital region is associated with sustained benefit over a 1-year period in some patients with CM, including some considered to have intractable disease.
- Patient-centered outcomes, such as quality of life, disability, and patient satisfaction, are important measures in PNS device trials in patients with CM.
- Although the surgical techniques associated with implantation of PNS devices for ONS have improved, the complication rates are still high, and refinements in both the technology and implantation techniques are required.

PRISM 2009 (Boston Scientific)

This study enrolled 132 patients. There was no statistically significant reduction in headache days with ONS versus sham. It was reported as an abstract only.

Numerous other studies are available in the literature for review. The measurement parameters and endpoints vary greatly; however, some generalizations and trends can be gleaned from the data. With the understanding that reported data vary according to indication, it appears that initial ONS responses are quite good, with up to 80% of patients continuing to use ONS at 1 year across various studies, although the continuation rate seems to drop to around 50–60% in case series with longer follow-ups, of varied duration. The short-term effectiveness of ONS appears to be maintained in patients who continue to use their devices.

Newer wireless SCS and PNS electrode devices have recently appeared on the market and are being used for a variety of peripheral neuropathy conditions including craniofacial pain. These do not require tunneling or an implanted IPG and are powered via an external antenna and battery system. Since the system remains in situ, there is the possibility that migration and infection will be significantly reduced.

Further Reading

Acar F, Miller J, Golshani KJ, Israel ZH, McCartney S, & Burchiel K. Pain relief after cervical ganglionectomy (C2 and C3) for the treatment of medically intractable occipital neuralgia. Stereotactic and Functional Neurosurgery. 2008;86(2):106–112. https://doi.org/10.1159/000113872

Brewer AC, Trentman T L, Ivancic MG, et al. Long-term outcome in occipital nerve stimulation patients with medically intractable primary headache disorders. Neuromodulation: Technology at the Neural Interface. 2013;16:557–564. doi:10.1111/j.1525-1403.2012.00490.x

Choi KS, Ko Y, Kim YS, et al. Long-term outcome and prognostic factors after C2 ganglion decompression in 68 consecutive patients with intractable occipital neuralgia. Acta Neurochir (Wien). 2015 Jan;157(1):85–89.

The International Classification of Headache Disorders, 3rd edition (beta version). Cephalalgia. 2016;33(9):629–808.

Jenkins B, Tepper SJ. Neurostimulation for primary headache disorders, Part 1: Pathophysiology and anatomy, history of neuromodulation in headache treatment, and review of *peripheral* neuromodulation in primary headaches. Headache: The Journal of Head and Face Pain. 2011;51:1254–1266.

Saper, JR, Dodick, DW, Silberstein, SD et al., ONSTIM Investigators. Occipital nerve stimulation for the treatment of intractable chronic migraine headache: ONSTIM feasibility study. Cephalalgia. 2011;31:271–285.

Palmisani S, Al-Kaisy A, Arcioni R, et al. A six year retrospective review of occipital nerve stimulation practice: controversies and challenges of an emerging technique for treating refractory headache syndromes. Journal of Headache and Pain. 2013;14:67. DOI: 10.1186/1129-2377-14-67

Sweet JA, Mitchell LS, Narouze, et al. Occipital nerve stimulation for the treatment of patients with medically refractory occipital neuralgia: congress of neurological surgeons systematic review and evidence-based guideline. Neurosurgery. 2015 Sep;77(3):332–341. doi: 10.1227/NEU.0000000000000872

Weiner RL, Reed KL. Peripheral neurostimulation for the control of intractable occipital neuralgia. Neuromodulation. 1999;2:369–375.

Geniculate Neuralgia

Emily Lehmann Levin

8

Case Presentation

A 44-year-old woman with no significant past medical history presents with a 1-year history of right ear pain. The pain is deep within the ear. She describes it as like an "ice pick" through her ear canal. It is episodic and she is free of pain between episodes. It initially started when cleaning her ears with a cotton swab. It now can come without provocation or with introduction of an object into the external auditory meatus. She initially presented to her primary care physician, who found no evidence of otitis media or otitis externa. She was then referred to her dentist for evaluation for temporomandibular joint dysfunction. An oral appliance provided no relief. Her dentist recommended evaluation by an otolaryngologist. There was no evidence of malignancy of the external ear. Audiometry was normal. She was started on carbamazepine with a significant improvement in the frequency and severity of attacks. She then developed severe hyponatremia, requiring discontinuation of the carbamazepine. Full neurologic examination is completely normal.

Questions

1. What is the likely diagnosis?
2. What diagnoses are important to exclude?
3. What is the most appropriate imaging modality?
4. What is the appropriate timing of further work-up?

Assessment and Planning

The neurosurgeon suspects the diagnosis of geniculate neuralgia. This diagnosis is supported by the patient's description of the pain, its location in the inner ear, the trigger point within the ear canal, and the periods of time without pain punctuated by lancinating episodes of pain, as well as the response to carbamazepine. Geniculate neuralgia may also be associated with disorders of lacrimation, gustatory sensation, and salivation. It is important to exclude other causes of inner ear pain, including dental dysfunction, inflammation or infection within the ear, or malignancy of the concha. It is also important to image the head and neck to identify any other lesions that may contribute. Deep ear pain may also be caused by glossopharyngeal or trigeminal neuralgia.

Glossopharyngeal neuralgia is typically associated with throat pain and triggered with swallowing, while trigeminal neuralgia involves a greater portion of the face.

The radiographic examination of choice in this case is an MRI with high resolution focused on the brainstem. This was completed and was notable for a small vascular structure in conflict with the CNVII/VIII complex (Figure 8.1). A CT of the neck was also normal.

Oral Boards Review—Diagnostic Pearls

1. Like trigeminal neuralgia, geniculate neuralgia is a clinical diagnosis, based on the description of the pain, its distribution, and the history of its evolution. Imaging only supplements and refines the diagnosis.
2. The physical examination of the patient with geniculate neuralgia is invariably normal. Any cranial nerve deficits should raise concern for lesional or secondary pain conditions.
3. Geniculate neuralgia is exceptionally rare, with fewer than 150 cases reported in the literature.

In this case, the patient described features consistent with geniculate neuralgia. The imaging studies were reassuring for the absence of mass lesions in the head or neck, and there was a suggestion of a vascular etiology inasmuch as the patient had a conflicting vessel on the symptomatic side.

Questions

1. How do these clinical and radiological findings influence surgical planning?
2. How would the absence of a neurovascular contact on the symptomatic side influence plans for surgery?

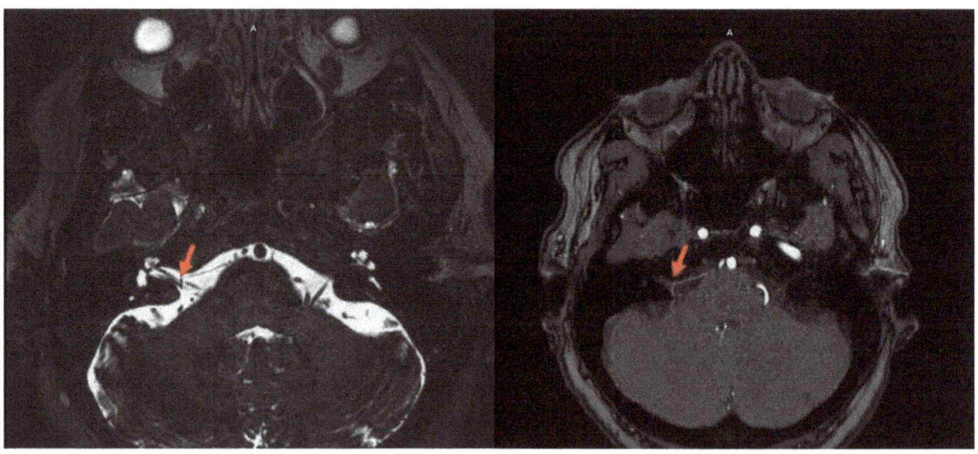

Figure 8.1. MRI FIESTA sequence (left) and MR angiography (right) demonstrating a small vascular structure in conflict with the right CNVII/VIII complex (red arrow).

Decision Making

Unlike the symptoms of trigeminal neuralgia, which present with pain in a clear sensory distribution, otalgic neuralgia may have involvement from multiple cranial nerves. The ear is innervated by branches of cranial nerves V, VII, IX, and X. Geniculate neuralgia is defined as intermittent episodes of pain located deep in the ear that last for seconds or minutes and are often triggered by sensory or mechanical stimuli at the posterior wall of the auditory canal, without any pathology. It is believed to originate from the nervus intermedius, so named because of its intermediate position between the facial nerve and the superior portion of the vestibular nerve. The nervus intermedius provides sensation to the concha of the auricle, the mastoid region, portions of the posterior wall of the external auditory canal, and the outer layer of the tympanic membrane. It also carries parasympathetic secretory fibers to the lacrimal, submandibular, and nasopalatine glands and sensory fibers from the gustatory nucleus. It is advisable to locate the trigger point for the neuralgia within the sensory territory of the nervus intermedius.

Medical therapy for geniculate neuralgia is similar to that for trigeminal neuralgia. Carbamazepine is the first-line therapy, along with gabapentin, lamotrigine, and tricyclic antidepressants. More advanced procedures may be considered in the event that medical therapy is ineffective or poorly tolerated. Much like trigeminal neuralgia, it is possible to perform a local blockade to anesthetize the trigger point to provide temporary relief as well as diagnostic guidance.

As it is relatively rare, there is little evidence supporting the best surgical treatment for geniculate neuralgia. A recent review has advocated for a retromastoid craniotomy for exploration of the cerebellopontine angle with microvascular decompression of any impingement on the root entry zone of cranial nerves VII, VIII, IX or X, along with sectioning of the nervus intermedius. This builds upon the work of Lovely and Jannetta, who published their series in 1997.

Surgical Procedure

Microvascular decompression/nervus intermedius sectioning is a major procedure carried out under general anesthetic with a Foley catheter in place, IV access and invasive arterial blood pressure monitoring. Brainstem auditory evoked responses are routinely used. Facial nerve monitoring and trigeminal nerve monitoring may also be performed.

Positioning and exposure for this procedure is similar to that for microvascular decompression for trigeminal neuralgia. Patients are positioned either semilateral or lateral, with the head placed in Mayfield pins and turned away from the operative side with the vertex angled toward the floor in order to improve the surgical angle to the lower cranial nerves. The ipsilateral shoulder is frequently taped caudally to improve the angle of visualization. Care should be taken to ensure that the brachial plexus is not overly stretched and that venous drainage through the neck is not compromised. The incision is centered on the asterion, and may be linear or "C" or "S" shaped. The angle of the transverse-sigmoid junction must be defined in the bony opening, allowing adequate access to the cerebellopontine angle. The exposure for a nervus intermedius operation is not fundamentally different from its trigeminal counterpart. Once the scalp is opened, the surgeon can perform either a craniotomy or a craniectomy, based on the sinus angle. The edges of the transverse and sigmoid sinuses should be seen after the bony removal is complete.

The size of the cranial opening is variable, but is usually around 3 cm in diameter. The bony edges should be waxed thoroughly to avoid cerebrospinal fluid (CSF) penetration into any mastoid air cells. The dura is opened and CSF is allowed to drain, until which point the cerebellum relaxes and CSF spontaneously drains from the opening. At this point, the surgeon gently retracts the lateral portion of the lateral cerebellar hemisphere, proceeding under high magnification along the petrous face, until the facial and vestibulocochlear nerve complex comes into view. Rhoton described the course of the nervus intermedius through the cistern and noted that, in approximately 20% of cases, it is impossible to identify the nerve as it is attached to the vestibular portion of the vestibulocochlear nerve. Typically, the nerve is positioned between the facial nerve and the superior portion of the vestibular nerve. The dissection is challenging. Careful attention to the degree of retraction placed on the facial and vestibulocochlear nerves is necessary to avoid complication, and neuromonitoring can assist with this. Brainstem auditory evoked potential monitoring is, therefore, the standard of care when performing this procedure.

Just caudal to the VII/VIII nerve complex the surgeon will find cranial nerves IX and X. Once these nerves are identified, the surgeon may explore the root entry zone of the glossopharyngeal nerve, addressing any compressive etiologies along the way in a manner similar to that for trigeminal neuralgia, placing Teflon pledgets in between each nerve and the impinging vascular loop.

Following the completion of the decompression and/or the nerve section, the dura is closed. The bone flap may be replaced, but this is not a necessity. The incision is closed tightly in layers to reduce the risk of CSF leak.

Oral Boards Review—Management Pearls

1. Positioning of the head with adequate turning to expose the retroauricular region, and a downward tilt of the head to improve the surgical angle, are important.
2. Brainstem Auditory Evoked Response (BAER) monitoring is necessary to reduce the risk of hearing loss with surgery, as cerebellar retraction may cause unrecognized stretching of the cochlear fibers.

Pivot Points

1. Imaging may point to a vascular compression etiology for the neuralgia, but the decision to perform a microvascular decompression (rather than a nerve section) should take into account other factors, such as patient age and comorbidities.
2. BAER monitoring during surgery is an important safeguard against excessive retraction.
3. Unlike trigeminal neuralgia, there are no percutaneous options for treatment.

Aftercare

Following the procedure, patients are typically monitored in the intensive care unit for the first 24 hours and may be discharged within a day or two. In order to lessen symptoms of aseptic meningitis, an oral steroid taper is often prescribed. Routine imaging is not necessary. Small pseudomeningoceles are not uncommon, and they usually resolve spontaneously.

Complications and Management

Complications specific to sectioning of the nervus intermedius include cessation of tearing on the ipsilateral eye and loss of taste on the anterior 2/3 of the tongue, though a number of patients did not report these issues post-operatively. Otherwise, the most frequent complication of exploration of the lower cranial nerves is aseptic meningitis, likely to be related to blood in the CSF or the presence of Teflon. Symptoms consist of headache, neck stiffness, and low-grade fever. This is often managed with a short course of steroids. Of course, one must consider septic meningitis. If there is significant fever or the patient appears more ill, a lumbar puncture is indicated.

This procedure may also be complicated by CSF rhinorrhea, usually related to CSF egress from the dural opening through a mastoid air cell into the middle ear and through the Eustachian tubes into the nasopharynx. When present, CSF rhinorrhea is relatively straightforward to manage, given the superficial nature of the CSF egress pathway. A lumbar drain may be placed temporarily to allow the hole in the mastoid air cell to seal, but if this does not resolve the issue, a superficial re-exploration, with resealing of the air cells will stop the leak.

Less frequent complications include hearing loss, facial paralysis, swallowing difficulties, hoarseness, or cerebellar infarction. Hearing loss may occur, especially in older patients. BAER monitoring is helpful to reduce the risk of this complication. If waveforms diminish during the surgical approach, it is advisable to temporarily cease manipulation and retraction and allow waveforms to recover before continuing. Facial paralysis is very unusual and is usually a sign of excessive retraction. It is frequently accompanied by significant hearing loss. Swallowing problems or hoarseness are distinctly uncommon. Cerebellar stroke is usually a sign of significant cerebellar retraction or suboptimal positioning at the start of surgery.

Oral Boards Review—Complications Pearls

1. Careful patient positioning is essential to improve visualization and reduce the need for cerebellar retraction during surgery, reducing the risk of the most serious complications of the operation.
2. The most common complications of MVD surgery, aseptic meningitis and CSF rhinorrhea, are relatively straightforward to manage.
3. BAER monitoring allows the surgeon to reduce tension on the facial and cochlear nerves, reducing the risk of cranial neuropathies as a result of surgery.

Evidence and Outcomes

As geniculate neuralgia is rare, there is little evidence to support the optimal surgical therapy. The case series that exist often did not use specific diagnostic criteria and included patients with atypical facial pain as well as pharyngeal pain. There was no systematic approach to treatment with most reporting decompression of multiple cranial nerves at the time of surgery, with or without sectioning of the nervus intermedius. Lovely and Jannetta reported patients in whom multiple procedures were performed where they were unable to achieve lasting pain relief until the nervus intermedius was sectioned. This limited evidence supports sectioning of the nervus intermedius when feasible along with decompression of obvious vascular compression of cranial nerves V, VII, VIII, IX, and X. Further studies would be helpful to determine optimal treatment.

Further Reading

1. Rhoton AL, Kobayashi S, Hollinshead WH. Nervus intermedius. *J Neurosurg*. 1968;29(6):609–618. doi:10.3171/jns.1968.29.6.0609
2. Tubbs RS, Steck DT, Mortazavi MM, Cohen-Gadol AA. The nervus intermedius: a review of its anatomy, function, pathology, and role in neurosurgery. *World Neurosurgery*. 2013;79(5-6):763–767. doi:10.1016/j.wneu.2012.03.023
3. Tubbs RS, Mosier KM, Cohen-Gadol AA. Geniculate neuralgia: clinical, radiologic, and intraoperative correlates. *World Neurosurgery*. 2013;80(6):e353–e357. doi:10.1016/j.wneu.2012.11.053.
4. Rupa V, Saunders RL, Weider DJ. Geniculate neuralgia: the surgical management of primary otalgia. *J Neurosurg*. 1991;75(4):505–511. doi:10.3171/jns.1991.75.4.0505
5. Lovely TJ, Jannetta PJ. Surgical management of geniculate neuralgia. *Am J Otol*. 1997;18(4):512–517.
6. Tang IP, Freeman SR, Kontorinis G, et al. Geniculate neuralgia: a systematic review. *J Laryngol Otol*. 2014;128(5):394–399. doi:10.1017/S0022215114000802

Dorsal Root Entry Zone Lesioning for Brachial Plexus Avulsion Pain

Daniel R. Cleary and Sharona Ben-Haim

9

Case Presentation

A 26-year-old man presents to clinic 9 months after a high-speed motorcycle crash complaining of persistent, severe right-sided arm pain. He reports that he had a prolonged course in the ICU due to a head injury, and he has been in a rehabilitation unit for nearly one year. Since waking up in the ICU, he noticed that his right arm didn't work as well as the left, as well as numbness in various regions of the arm. After his injury, he also developed progressively worsening pain throughout the arm, which has become intolerable. Upon discharge, he was told that he has recovered fully from his head injury, and that an MRI showed no injury to his spinal cord. His doctors at the time told him he had "nerve injury" in his right arm, and that he did not require surgery.

Upon presentation, he reports that he is frustrated that after months in rehabilitation, he is still having intractable pain. Furthermore, due to the combination of motor and sensory deficits, he is not able to use his right arm functionally. He has tried lidocaine patches, anti-convulsants, and acetaminophen without relief. He is currently on a regimen of gabapentin, tizanidine, oxycodone, and oxycontin, which are managed by a pain specialist. He complains that while the medications make him groggy, he cannot function without them due to frequent bursts of shooting, electrical pain and a constant burning sensation. He was referred to neurosurgery clinic to explore further pain management options. He has also considered amputation of the arm as a possible solution.

Exam of the right arm and forearm reveals atrophy of both extensors and flexors. He is able to abduct his shoulder with 3/5 strength, he is able flex his elbow with 2/5 strength, but he cannot extend the elbow, has no flexion or extension at the wrist, and cannot flex, extend, or abduct his fingers. He reports diminished sensation at the shoulder, numbness along the extensor surfaces of the arm, forearm, and both sides of the hand, but he has preserved but significantly diminished sensation along the flexor surface of the arm and proximal forearm. The patient reports severe pain throughout the entire arm and forearm characterized by a painful sensitivity to light touch and 3 to 4 episodes of spontaneous shooting pain throughout the arm during the day. At this time, he rates his pain at 6/10 while at rest.

> **Questions**
>
> 1. What is the differential diagnosis?
> 2. What anatomical injury is most likely to account for the patient's pain?

3. What is the most appropriate imaging modality to confirm diagnosis?
4. Why would amputation not improve the patient's pain?
5. What are the most likely affected levels?
6. What additional neurophysiological studies would be of benefit for surgical planning?

Assessment and Planning

The patient is a candidate for an ablative procedure for the treatment of his pain. The most likely diagnosis is brachial plexus stretch injury or root avulsion. Motorcycle riders are especially susceptible to brachial plexus injury and nerve root avulsion, which occurs when the shoulder is violently driven in an opposing direction from the head and neck, such as with a high-speed ejection and landing directly on the chest and shoulder.

A thin-cut MRI is obtained of the patient's cervical spine, which shows no evidence of central cord injury, but does show evidence of root disruption at C6 and T1 and cyst formation at the C7 and C8 root entry zones, consistent with pseudomeningocele. A needle electromyelograph shows decreased motor amplitude and conduction velocity in the deltoid and biceps with low amplitude voluntary motor potentials, but an absence of motor potentials in the brachioradialis, triceps, extensor digitorum communis, first dorsal interosseus, and abductor policis brevis. Fibrillations were not seen. Sensory conduction studies show decreased amplitude and conduction velocity in the C5 dermatome, and significantly diminished sensory nerve action potentials in the insensate dermatomes. Interpretation of the results suggests a stretch injury to C5 with chronic, pre-ganglionic avulsion of the nerve roots at C6, C7, C8, and T1.

The imaging and neurophysiological findings are shared with the patient, and the surgeon explains that amputation would not be likely to improve the pain, because the nerves appear to have already been disconnected from the spinal cord and are not transmitting signals effectively. Options for treatment are discussed with the patient, including both continued conservative management and neurosurgical intervention. The operative intervention recommended is a dorsal root entry zone (DREZ) lesion, or DREZotomy, to the affected levels of the spinal cord.

Questions

1. Are patients more likely to develop post-avulsion pain from pre- or post-ganglionic avulsion?
2. Would a nerve repair or nerve graft have prevented the patient's current problems?
3. What is the difference between neuropathic pain and nociceptive pain?

Decision Making

Surgical treatment for extremity pain depends on the underlying pathology. Ablation of the dorsal root entry zone (DREZ lesioning or DREZotomy) is a technique that developed following previous failures to effectively control pain resulting from brachial plexus avulsion. The goal of DREZotomy is the destruction of second-order neurons in Rexed lamina II (substantia gelatinosa), which are largely nociceptive specific. Nerve root avulsion removes the dorsal root ganglia, but the second-order neurons in the spinal cord and their ascending afferent connections are preserved. In the absence of peripheral input, these dorsal horn neurons can develop increased firing and hyperactivity. Thus, ablation of these second-order neurons can eliminate the increased ascending signaling. DREZotomy is an effective treatment for neuropathic pain secondary to brachial plexus avulsion and end-zone spinal cord injury pain, and may also be effective in post-herpetic syndrome and spasticity.

Oral Boards Review—Diagnostic Pearls

- The surgical treatment of pain requires knowledge of the functional neuroanatomy underlying nociceptive signal transmission and of the changes in the nervous system with chronic pain. Terminology is also important: "nociception" refers to the objective detection of tissue damage, "pain" refers to discomfort from the subjective experience of real or imagined injury, and "neuropathic" refers to the perception of pain with or without tissue damage due to injury to the nervous system.
- In the uninjured nervous system, peripheral receptors in the skin detect subtle changes in pressure and temperature. In the transition from innocuous to noxious stimulation, additional receptors are recruited, including nociceptors, responsible for the evaluation of impending or actual tissue damage. Tissue damage releases a "soup" of neurotransmitters, including bradykinins, prostaglandins, serotonin, and histamine, which recruits additional receptors and potentiates the already excited nerve endings. The signals from the nociceptive fibers are transmitted through the peripheral nerves to the dorsal root ganglion, which then primarily synapse in laminae I, II, and V of the dorsal horn. Nociceptive second-order neurons in the dorsal horn extend axons across the midline either at the level of entry or at one to two levels above or below. These axons join other fibers to become the spinothalamic tract, which ascends on the ventral and the ventrolateral surfaces of the spinal cord to synapse in the contralateral thalamus.
- A distinct spinal pathway exists for nociceptive transmission, but other pathways may be recruited in neuropathic or chronic pain, which makes surgical treatment more difficult. Targeted lesions have been attempted at all levels of the nervous system, with mixed results. For instance, neurectomy or rhizotomy may effectively relieve acute pain by producing anesthesia in the affected distribution but is ineffective for deafferentation or neuropathic pain, and patients may eventually develop rebound neuropathic pain. Lesions to the spinothalamic tract (cordotomy) provide effective relief for inflammatory or malignancy-related pain, but the technique is not effective for deafferentation or neuropathic pain, which suggests that alternative pathways may develop in abnormal pain states. DREZ lesioning is one of the few techniques that provides effective relief of neuropathic and other pathological pain states.

Pre-operative evaluation of the pain patient should take into account the etiology of the injury, the nature and character of the pain, the chronicity of the injury, and the psychological profile of the patient. Importantly, the surgeon should impress realistic expectations upon the patient pre-operatively, noting that the procedure may not provide immediate relief, may only provide partial relief, and that the pain may recur in months to years. Additionally, complicating factors such as chronic opioid use may dramatically affect the patient's perception of relief from pain.

Despite the emotional distress caused by the pain, the timing of the procedure is largely elective, and the patient should be medically optimized for surgery prior to the procedure. However, providers should be alert for suicidal ideation or planning in patients expressing an inability to cope with their pain.

Questions

1. What spinal tract is immediately medial to the dorsal horn?
2. What significant motor spinal tract lies lateral to the dorsal horn
3. Where do the nerve rootlets enter the spinal cord?

Surgical Procedure

Ablation of the dorsal horn of the spinal cord is a major operation with significant risks and should be carried out by experienced surgeons. Prior to the procedure, the patient should be appropriately informed of the risks and benefits.

Much of the setup is similar to that of a cervical hemi-laminectomy, but additional requirements include neurophysiological monitoring (somatosensory-evoked potentials, motor-evoked potentials, and a stimulation probe), microscopy, fluoroscopy, and surgeon's preference of tool for ablation (sharp bipolar, radio-frequency probe, or ultrasonic probe). Anesthesia induction may use relaxation, but maintenance should not include paralytics, and a motor baseline is necessary.

The patient is placed in a 3-pin head holder and positioned prone on chest rolls with the head slightly flexed forward ("Concord position"). The hips and knees should be slightly flexed and the bed placed in reverse Trendelenburg to allow for a relaxed operating position while minimizing venous congestion. A midline incision is made and the dissection is carried down along the intermuscular raphe until the spinous process are encountered. The ipsilateral laminae are exposed, taking care not to disrupt the facets laterally or the interspinous ligament medially. Fluoroscopy is important for localization, but it is important to note that bony anatomy will not necessarily correspond to the locations of the rootlets. For instance, in avulsion of C5 to T1, bony exposure of C3 to C7 is sufficient for the procedure. After an appropriate hemilaminectomy is performed, the dura is opened and the dorsolateral sulcus identified by the entry of the dorsal rootlets. In cases of complete avulsion, the anatomy may be distorted by the absence of rootlets, cord atrophy, arachnoid adhesions, or gliosis. Care should be taken in freeing adhesions and identifying appropriate levels. Electrical stimulation is essential for identifying the appropriate levels; stimulation at C4 should cause diaphragm movement, whereas stimulation at other levels should evoke peripheral responses in the appropriate muscle groups (where maintained). Areas for ablation should include any nearby dermatomes where the patient has pain.

Oral Boards Review—Management Pearls

- Knowledge of the microscopic spinal anatomy is essential when performing cervical DREZotomy. The dorsal rootlets enter the spinal cord through the dorsolateral sulcus, and Lissauer's tract is the continuation of the fibers en route to the dorsal horn. The dorsal horn is divided into 10 layers (the Rexed laminae), with layer 2 being most involved in nociception, and the deeper laminae III, IV, and V primarily processing other sensory aspects. Laminae VII in the thoracic cord contains the intermediolateral nucleus, which mediates sympathetic innervation. Layers VIII and IX in the cervical cord contains motor interneurons and motor neurons, including neurons that that control the phrenic nerve.
- Two major spinal tracts border the dorsal horn: medially is the fasciculus cuneatus and laterally is the lateral corticospinal tract. The fasciculus cuneatus is located in the lateral segment of the dorsal columns, and it is composed of sensory afferents that transmit light-touch, vibration, and proprioception. The corticospinal tract is the dominant descending motor pathway, composed of fibers that originate in the motor cortex and synapse onto lower motor neurons in the spinal cord. Damage to either of these tracts may result in new sensory and motor deficits.

Once the dorsal root entry zone at the appropriate level is identified, the dorsolateral sulcus is opened sharply with a microknife knife at approximately 30 degrees from midline to a depth of 1–2 mm. The most common lesioning methods are sharp bipolar cautery or radiofrequency ablation, but ultrasonic ablation, laser ablation, and aspiration have been used with varying degrees of success. Under direct microscopic visualization, the appropriate tool is inserted to a depth of 3 mm from the surface of the cord at a 30-degree angle, and the dorsal horn is ablated. The process is repeated in the affected areas at a separation of approximately 1 mm, which may require 50–60 lesions. The use of impedance measurements may help determine the appropriate placement and depth. Special care should be taken to avoid coagulating surface arterioles or other vessels. After completion, the dura should be closed in a watertight fashion, and the incision should be closed in layers in standard fashion. A surgical drain is useful if there is concern for CSF leak.

Pivot Point

- Outcomes of DREZotomy depend in part on the character of the pain. Paroxysmal, allodynic, and deafferentation pain respond well to DREZ, whereas constant pain has a lower response rate. If the patient may not substantially benefit from the procedure, the surgeon and patient should have an in-depth discussion as to whether the projected benefits are worth the surgical risks, and whether a different procedure or continued medical management would be more appropriate.

Aftercare

Post-operative care should be similar to that of a laminotomy or multilevel hemilaminectomy. Drain placement and duration is at the discretion of the operating physician. Patients should be maintained on their current pain regimen, with an appropriate increase for post-operative pain. If available, a pain management consulting service should be enlisted for in-patient management of patient's regimen and outpatient weaning of medications.

Complications and Management

Complications may be divided into routine complications from spine surgery and specific complications related to the ablation. Standard approach-related complications include pain, wound breakdown, wound infection, CSF leak, and meningitis, which should be managed in the usual fashion. Surgeons should be aware of the long-term risk of post-laminectomy cervical kyphosis, and care should be taken not to disrupt the facets or the interspinous ligaments.

Complications specific to the ablative procedure stem from inadvertent injury to the nearby structures within the cord. Medial and lateral to the dorsal horn are the dorsal columns and the corticospinal tracts, respectively. Distorted anatomy including arachnoid adhesions or cord atrophy may result in inappropriate lesion placement and lead to post-operative motor or sensory deficits.

Oral Boards Review—Complications Pearls

- Minimal hemilaminectomy without disruption of nearby spinal structures will reduce risk of post-laminectomy cervical kyphosis
- Upper extremity, unilateral sensory deficits may result from damage to nearby fasciculus cuneatus, which is medial to the dorsal horn. Similarly, upper extremity, unilateral motor deficits may result from damage to corticospinal tract, which is lateral. A large lesion or a greater degree of misplacement may also result in deficits in the lower extremity.

Evidence and Outcomes

In the right population, DREZotomy is one of the most efficacious neurosurgical procedures for pain, and has excellent long-term outcomes. No randomized trials have been performed on DREZ lesions for brachial plexus injury, but a number of retrospective and fewer prospective studies describe a high percentage of patients with continued pain relief several years after the surgery.

Thomas and Kitchen (1994) reported results for 44 patients who underwent DREZ lesion for brachial plexus injury at an average of 5 years follow-up. Of these patients, 77% reported "good" or "fair" pain control, although 18% of patients had persistent neurological deficit. In a case series of 19 patients with 4.9 years average follow-up, Awad et al. (2013) reported that 69% of patients who had DREZ had continued "excellent" or "good" pain control, and 84% of patients would go through the procedure again. In another series, Chen and Tu (2006) reported similar findings: Of 60 cases of DREZ lesion for brachial plexus avulsion, 80% of patients had "excellent" or "good" pain relief in the early post-op period, although the rate dropped to 60% at 5 years and 50% at 10 years. Aichaoui et al (2011) reported on a series of 29 patients who underwent DREZ for brachial plexus injury, with emphasis on control by pain characteristic. For paroxysmal pain, 85% of patients report "good" or "excellent" control, whereas for constant pain only 73% of patients reported control.

Further Reading

Aichaoui, F., Mertens, P., & Sindou, M. (2011). Dorsal root entry zone lesioning for pain after brachial plexus avulsion: results with special emphasis on differential effects on the paroxysmal versus the continuous components. A prospective study in a 29-patient consecutive series. *PAIN®*, *152*(8), 1923–1930.

Awad, A. J., Forbes, J. A., Jermakowicz, W., Eli, I. M., Blumenkopf, B., & Konrad, P. (2013). Experience with 25 years of dorsal root entry zone lesioning at a single institution. *Surgical Neurology International*, *4*, 64.

Chen, H. J., & Tu, Y. K. (2006). Long term follow-up results of dorsal root entry zone lesions for intractable pain after brachial plexus avulsion injuries. In J. W. Chang, Y. Katayama, & T. Yamamoto (Eds.), *Advances in Functional and Reparative Neurosurgery* (pp. 73–75). Vienna: Springer.

Friedman, A. H., & Bullitt, E. (1988). Dorsal root entry zone lesions in the treatment of pain following brachial plexus avulsion, spinal cord injury and herpes zoster. *Stereotactic and Functional Neurosurgery*, *51*(2-5), 164–169.

Nashold Jr., B. S., & Ostdahl, R. H. (1979). Dorsal root entry zone lesions for pain relief. *Journal of Neurosurgery*, *51*(1), 59–69.

Samii, M., Bear-Henney, S., Lüdemann, W., Tatagiba, M., & Blömer, U. (2001). Treatment of refractory pain after brachial plexus avulsion with dorsal root entry zone lesions. *Neurosurgery*, *48*(6), 1269–1277.

Sindou, M. (1988). DREZ lesions for brachial plexus injury. *Neurosurgery*, *23*(4), 528.

Sindou, M. P., Blondet, E., Emery, E., & Mertens, P. (2005). Microsurgical lesioning in the dorsal root entry zone for pain due to brachial plexus avulsion: a prospective series of 55 patients. *Journal of Neurosurgery*, *102*(6), 1018–1028.

Thomas, D. G., & Kitchen, N. D. (1994). Long-term follow up of dorsal root entry zone lesions in brachial plexus avulsion. *Journal of Neurology, Neurosurgery & Psychiatry*, *57*(6), 737–738.

Percutaneous Cordotomy for Cancer-Associated Pain

Marian M. Bercu, Timothy Shepherd, and Alon Y. Mogilner

10

Case Presentation

A 70-year-old male was referred by his pain-management physician for intervention. Five years prior, the patient was diagnosed with adenocarcinoma of the esophagus with positive lymph node involvement. He was treated by esophagectomy, chemotherapy and intensity-modulated radiation therapy at a later time due to local recurrence. Further follow-up revealed new liver metastases, as well as several subcentimeter pulmonary lesions, and the patient was treated with a monoclonal antibody (ramucirumab). Routine PET/CT (positron emission/computed tomography) evaluation was consistent with disease progression, including a new paraspinal soft tissue mass, posterior to the initial gastroesophageal anastomosis, consistent with well-differentiated adenocarcinoma per needle biopsy, treated by stereotactic radiosurgery.

During the year prior to presentation, the patient started complaining of gradually increasing pain involving the right scapula, across the chest toward the sternum and the right shoulder with radiation to the elbow and wrist. The pain was constant and stabbing pain in the shoulder and chest areas and burning in the arm. He rated it 10/10 and it was aggravated by any type of touch. Multiple medication trials were attempted, with minimal relief. Current regimen included gabapentin and methadone, which were providing minimal benefit, and their use was complicated by multiple side effects (especially somnolence and constipation). The pain affected the patient's quality of life, restricting all his activities, and resulting in severe depression. A cervical epidural steroid injection failed to provide any further benefits. On exam, he was cachectic in severe discomfort with obvious depressive features. No focal motor or sensory findings were noted, except for diffuse weakness and pain in the previously described distribution.

Questions

1. What is the likely diagnosis?
2. What is the most appropriate imaging modality?
3. What interventions would most benefit the patient?

Assessment and Planning

The functional neurosurgeon suspects a metastatic lesion involving or in the vicinity of the cervico-thoracic region. The main differential diagnosis may include a brachial plexus lesion; however, the extent of the dermatomes involved is not highly consistent with such a finding. A central lesion, for example a metastasis involving the thalamus, might be suspected as well.

In patients with metastatic cancer, one of most used imaging modalities is PET/CT, which can provide reliable information on the existence of new lesions; however, most central nervous system/peripheral nervous system lesions should be further evaluated by magnetic resonance imaging (MRI). Only when an MRI is contraindicated (e.g., in patients with implanted non-MRI compatible implants) or when bone-involving lesions need to be evaluated should a CT (computed tomography; usually with contrast) be performed.

Questions

1. What would be a relative contraindication to perform an MRI in this patient?
2. What MRI findings would require an additional cervico-thoracic CT (especially with thin-cut slices)?
3. What is a major consideration regarding the patient's disease status in relation to the extent of a planned surgical procedure?

Decision Making

The cervico-thoracic MRI revealed a large paravertebral mass, spanning from T5 to C6, infiltrating the right T2–4 lateral foramina. No bone involvement was noted. Given the location and size of the lesion, the patient's disease systemic status, and his prognosis, any resective surgical intervention aimed at alleviating his symptoms would have been contraindicated due to its extent, morbidity, and limited chances to provide pain relief. Patients who cannot be effectively managed by oral medications due to suboptimal efficacy or who suffer from significant side effects are candidates for procedures aimed to improve the pain control, such as intrathecal delivery systems or destructive procedures such as cordotomy.[1] The best candidates for a cordotomy procedure are patients with unilateral nociceptive-type somatic intractable pain secondary to malignancy[2] (Table 10.1).

Oral Boards Review—Diagnostic Pearls

1. PET/CT is useful in following cancer. Magnetic resonance supplies further details while CT provides bony details.
2. Intrathecal therapy and ablative lesions are main stays of cancer pain therapy treatment when oral opioids fail.
3. Currently open cordotomy is rare, and most procedures are performed in intraoperative CT or diagnostic CT suite.

Questions

1. What is the most common current approach for cordotomy?
2. What adjunct imaging should be used during the procedure?
3. What complication may occur after bilateral procedures?

Table 10.1: Summary of ideal patient for cordotomy, contraindications, and specific additional material risks to the procedure

Ideal Patient	Contraindications	Additional Risk
Unilateral nociceptive pain from extremity	Bilateral upper extremity pathology	Ondine's curse (apnea during sleep) if bilateral ablation
pO_2 > 80% on room air	Severe pulmonary dysfunction	Insufficient reserve to tolerate decreased function
Life expectancy between 3 and 12 mo	Survival < 3 mo or > 12 mo	Deafferentation pain > 6 mo after procedure
Normal ICP	Intracranial metastases and/or mass effect	Brain herniation during procedure
Absence of psychiatric comorbidities	Opiate dependence or emotional problems	Persistent pain control problems after cordotomy
Intact autonomic system	Sympathetic dysfunction*	Hypotension, Horner syndrome, bladder dysfunction
Comfortable in supine position	Orthopnea*	Inability to be supine long enough to complete procedure

Note: pO_2 indicates partial pressure of oxygen; ICP, intracranial pressure
* Relative contraindication.

Surgical Procedure

CT-guided percutaneous cervical cordotomy is an ablative procedure targeting the lateral spinothalamic tract in the anterolateral spinal cord. Somatic sensory signals are conveyed along two major ascending systems in the spinal cord: the anterolateral system and the dorsal column-medial lemniscal system.[3,4] The former carries information mainly related to pain and temperature, as well as some tactile information (Figure 10.1).

The axons of second order neurons decussate over 2 to 5 segments before entering the anterolateral columns. The system transmits sensory information predominantly to the contralateral thalamus and cortex; however, a minority of fibers also projects ipsilaterally. The cordotomy procedure aims to interrupt the ascending spinothalamic tract contralateral to the painful side; however, because of the high variability in the decussation level, ipsilateral analgesia may result. The spinothalamic tract in the anterolateral quadrant is organized somatotopically with the sacral segments posterolaterally, the leg anteromedially, and the arm and upper chest region fibers further anteromedially.

Although our practice is to perform the procedure in the radiology department CT suite, it can alternatively be performed in an operating room using an intra-operative CT.[5] In this case, the patient was brought into the CT suite and given intravenous sedation, under continuous anesthesia monitoring. We performed a cervical myelogram for the purpose of injecting contrast in the intrathecal space.[6] In addition, a CT angiogram of the skull base and upper cervical region was performed to evaluate for the presence of abnormal or aberrant vessels.

Next, the patient was placed in the right decubitus position with his head and neck flexed. A safe corridor for cisternal puncture was identified, cleaned, and draped in a sterile fashion. The skin and subcutaneous soft tissues were anesthetized with 1% lidocaine solution. A 9 cm 22-gauge spinal needle was inserted into the thecal space under

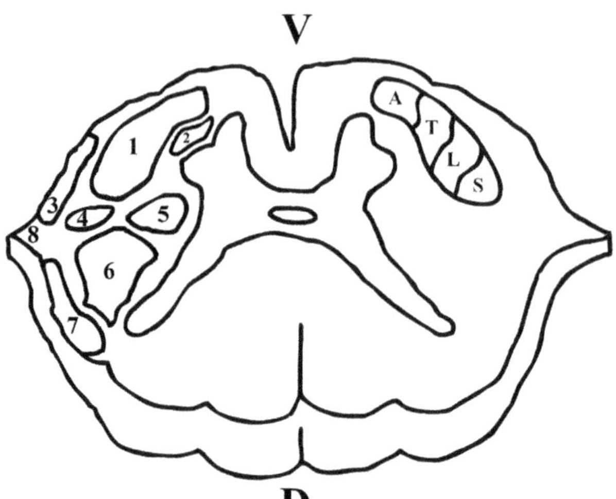

Figure 10.1. Schematic for the relevant functional anatomy of the axial cervical spinal cord when performing C1–2 cordotomy (V indicates ventral; and D, dorsal). Important ventral and lateral white matter pathways include the lateral spinothalamic tract (1), ventral reticulospinal tract (2), ventral spinocerebellar tract (3), lateral reticulospinal tract (4), rubrospinal tract (5), lateral corticospinal tract (6), dorsal spinocerebellar tract (7), and dentate ligament (8). Furthermore, it is important to understand the somatopic organization of the lateral spinothalamic tract delineated on the opposite side. A indicates arm; T, trunk; L, leg; and S, sacrum.

Source: Mogilner AY. Palliative CT-Guided Cordotomy for Medically Intractable Pain in Patients with Cancer. *AJNR Am J Neuroradiol* 2016;38:387–390. Reprinted with permission of the American Society of Neuroradiology.

intermittent CT image guidance. Upon confirmation of clear CSF return, approximately 8 mL of Omnipaque 300 contrast were injected slowly under intermittent CT guidance into the thecal space. The patient was rotated in multiple positions to redistribute contrast at the craniocervical junction over a 10-minute period, then replaced on the CT scanner in supine position with the head in a neutral position.

A left lateral C1-2 puncture with a standard 20-gauge spinal needle was performed, with the needle directed toward the anteromedial aspect of the cervical spinal cord as visualized by the CT myelogram of the cervical spine. Once CSF was obtained, axial CT scanning performed in-plane with the needle confirmed the trajectory as appropriate, aiming toward a point in the anterolateral quadrant of the cord approximately 2 mm anterior to the dentate ligament which would cover the arm and chest wall.

At that point, the cordotomy electrode (Cosman Medical, Burlington, Massachusetts) was then inserted so that the tip protruded by approximately 3 mm. Continued impedance monitoring was performed. The needle and electrode were then advanced slowly as the impedance jumped from 200 Ohms (consistent with CSF environment) to approximately 700 to 800 Ohms, indicating placement within the spinal cord (impedance is < 200 Ohms for CSF, < 400 Ohms for pail surface, and > 700 Ohms for cord parenchyma). CT scanning performed subsequently confirmed appropriate placement of the needle (Figure 10.2).

Following withdrawal of sedation, sensory and motor testing were performed. Stimulation began using a rate of 100 Hz (recommended range: 50–100 Hz) and pulse

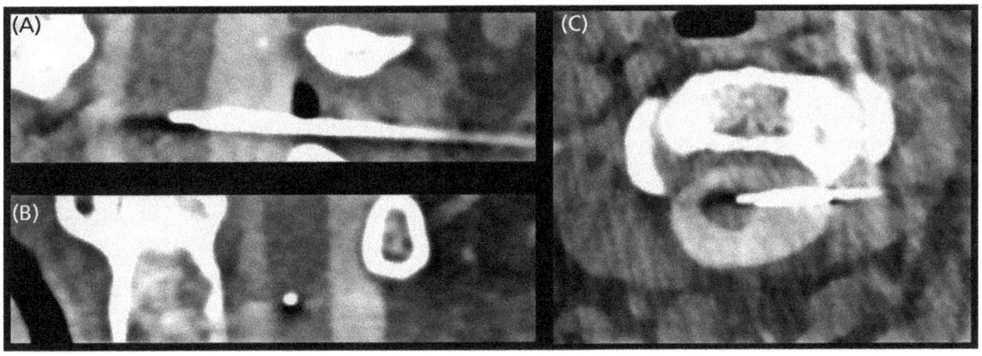

Figure 10.2. Coronal (A), sagittal (B), and axial (C) reformats of the CT myelogram demonstrate outer needle and inner electrode placement immediately before completion of a left lateral C1–2 cordotomy via radiofrequency ablation. The outer needle was placed into the thecal space near the pial surface of the cord approximately 2 mm ventral to the dentate ligament. The electrode was then advanced into the CSF, pia mater, and spinal cord with real-time monitoring of dynamic electrical impedance changes. Multimodal data, including the CT images, confirmed that the electrode was in the left spinothalamic tract. Note that the upper cervical cord is displaced to the right (an observation seen in multiple previous cases).

width of 0.1 msec. The voltage was slowly increased and at 0.15 V, the patient reported paresthesias in the right arm and chest wall (effect normally reported at 0.1–1.5 V). He denied any paresthesias in the leg. For further confirmation, motor testing was performed at a rate of 2 Hz and up to 1 V without noticing any contractions of the arm or leg (low frequency motor stimulation at 2–5 Hz, 0.2–1.5 V ideally does not provoke a motor response). Minimal ipsilateral trapezius contractions were noted at approximately 0.7 volts, which were expected. Significant trapezius contractions at low voltages may suggest that the electrode tip is too deep, stimulating the ventral horn neurons. Ipsilateral lower extremity movements indicate that the electrode is too posterior in the corticospinal tract. Thus, appropriate location of the electrode was confirmed.

A test lesion was made at 60 degrees centigrade for 60 seconds with no untoward effects. The patient's motor and sensory functions were re-examined, with no deficits noted. The sedation was restarted at a low level, and two lesions at 80 degrees for 60 seconds were performed. At the conclusion, the patient had no motor or new sensory deficits. The needle and the stylet were removed and a sterile dressing was applied. He was taken to the recovery room and discharged home following a two-hour monitoring interval, reporting significant improvement in his pain.

Oral Boards Review—Management Pearls

1. Percutaneous cordotomy should be considered as a first-line intervention in patients with refractory unilateral extremity pain secondary to malignancy
2. Test lesions should be performed and no adverse effects documented prior to full lesion under sedation.

Pivot Points

1. Unexpected motor side effects with stimulation may confirm suboptimal placement of the lead.
2. Significant trapezius contractions at low voltages suggest that the electrode tip is too deep.
3. Ipsilateral lower extremity movements indicate that the electrode is too posterior in the corticospinal tract.

Aftercare

In our experience, patients report immediate relief in their symptoms. Early in our treatments, the patients were discharged the following day. We monitored the patients for changes in pain control, limb strength or ataxia, respiratory status, and bowel or bladder functions. In recent cases, based on the previous safety and lack of complications, the patients could be safely discharged home the same day, as in this case after 2 hours of close monitoring, with routine precautions regarding possible post procedural headaches or the development of new neurological deficits. Any anticoagulation medications should be discontinued around the timing of the procedure, as per protocol of any neurosurgical intervention (Figure 10.3).

Complications and Management

Patients usually report immediate pain relief which is persistent after anesthesia wears off, as was in this case. We have not encountered any immediate or delayed complications or unexpected side effects. The classical complications of the procedure include respiratory insufficiency, headache, mirror pain, dysesthesia, and motor weakness.[8] Hemiparesis (ipsilateral) may occur, being irreversible in up to 8% of the cases in some series. In a large series presented by Kanpolat et al.,[11] of the 193 patients who underwent CT-guided

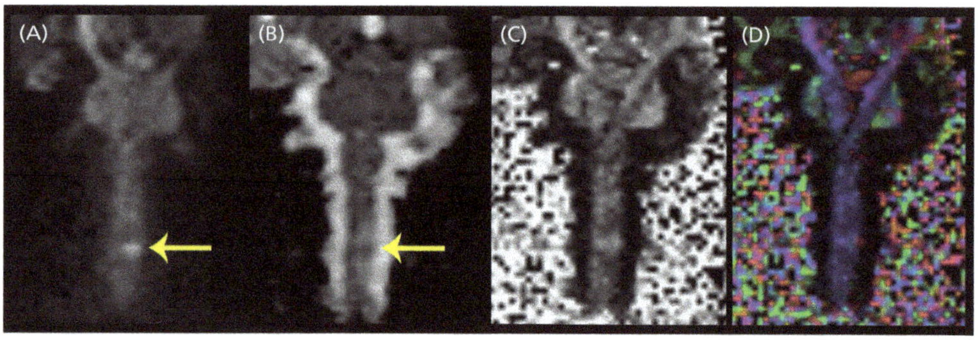

Figure 10.3. Coronal diffusion trace (A), apparent diffusion coefficient (B), fractional anisotropy (C), and color-encoded fractional anisotropy maps (D) of the cervical cord 48 hours after technically successful CT-guided left C1–2 cordotomy. There is a small focus of hyperintensity on the diffusion trace image with corresponding reduced diffusion indicative of focal cytotoxic edema (*arrow*) and more extensive surrounding vasogenic edema.

percutaneous cordotomy for cancer pain, the incidence of temporary motor dysfunction and ataxia was low (2.4%). Headaches as a result of the procedure are temporary in nature, as well as most of the dysesthetic syndromes (experienced by 2% of patients in the previously mentioned large series).

As previously reported by Krieger and Rosomoff et al. (mainly in the early years of performing the procedure over 45 years ago), respiratory dysfunction can be fatal, especially in bilateral procedures. Therefore, it is recommended to monitor those patients carefully, especially in the setting of pre-existing respiratory dysfunction. The exact mechanism of this complication is not well understood; however, it is partially related to the fact that fibers concerned with respiration run adjacent to the lateral spinothalamic tract in the anterolateral spinal cord down to the C3 level. If bilateral lesions are made, and those tracts are affected, a fatal sleep-induced apnea may be elicited (Ondine's curse or central hypoventilation syndrome). Patients after a pneumonectomy or other pulmonary insufficiency may succumb to this complication after only a unilateral lesion. This impairment may be identified by a pathologic hypercapnea challenge test result. It is imperative to mention the importance of the close follow up required from a pain management specialist.

Oral Boards Review—Complications Pearls

1. This procedure can be performed safely in experienced hands.
2. Post-procedure headache and recurrent pain are most common complications.
3. Bilateral procedures should be undertaken with great care.

Evidence and Outcomes

Percutaneous cordotomy was initially described by Müllan in 1963 as a development of the open cordotomy technique first reported by Schüller in 1910 and performed by Martin on January 19, 1911. Subsequently, the technique was further developed in parallel to the improvement to the imaging modalities, as well as the ablative technologies. The development of more potent oral medications together with intrathecal delivery systems, as well as the spinal cord stimulators, significantly reduced the number of such procedures in developed countries. Existing data for cordotomy is consistent with a relatively high success rate in carefully selected patients presenting with minimal side effects and low complication profile. However, the number of the procedures remained limited, as well as the available expertise outside major medical centers. It is important to emphasize that the duration of the procedure can be very short in experienced hands, and that the economic burden is significantly lower than that of an implantable neuromodulatory system, such as an intrathecal delivery system.

A prospective review of 45 patients treated by cordotomy, published in 2013 by Bain et al., shows a significant reduction from baseline in pain scores at 2 days and maintained through day 28 after the procedure. In this series, 35 patients presented with a mixed picture of both neuropathic and nociceptive pain, with a majority of 32 patients suffering from mesothelioma (19) and bronchial cancer (13) and reporting significant chest wall pain. In the mesothelioma subgroup, 9 of the 13 patients who were still under follow-up at day 28 reported a pain score of 0. Another interesting result is that at 28 days after the procedure, 39 out of 45 patients reported that the procedure was worthwhile. Post-procedural headaches were observed in 20 patients over a period of a couple of days only. At 28 days, 8 patients reported mirror pain; 1 patient reported an increase in his original pain, and persistent dysesthesia in another. There were no reported cases of bladder or bowel problems (rare complications, usually temporary, previously reported in small numbers, probably following mostly bilateral cordotomies). In 2008, Raslan reported a series of 41 patients treated by percutaneous cordotomy, with almost half suffering from chest wall pain due to mesothelioma.[7] At one month, 80% of the patients reported no pain. At six months follow up, 32% of patients reported no pain, with an additional 48% reporting partial but satisfactory pain relief.

The incidence of new pain following cordotomy is well-recognized (ranging from 6.5% to over 70%). In a series of 45 patients with unilateral pain who underwent CT-guided cordotomy, 33 patients (73.3%) reported new pain.[9] Further analysis of the etiology indicated that in 8 patients, the new pain was corresponding to pathological conditions of tissue such as tumor progression, while in 5 patients it was referred pain, but neither of these causes were identified in 15 patients. The new pain was in a mirror-image location in 28 patients and rostral to the original pain in 5 patients. The pain was temporary only in 7 patients and weaker than the original in 25 cases. The pathophysiological mechanisms underlying the development of new pain are not entirely understood. Experimental studies have shown that anterolateral spinal lesions result in behavioral hyperalgesia and dorsal horn hyperexcitability to noxious stimuli applied ipsilaterally to segments caudal to the lesion.[10] This effect is probably due to interruption of descending inhibitory systems. As previously reported by Fields and Basbaum, the interruption of the nociceptive input following a successful cordotomy appears to diminish activity in descending inhibitory systems. Contralateral referred pain, especially in a mirror-image location, may result from the activation of contralateral nociceptive spinal neurons through either direct commissural connections or supraspinal loops, as some experimental studies indicate. An abrupt decrease in the opioid medications following cordotomy might further enhance these mechanisms.

In conclusion, percutaneous cordotomy should be considered as a first-line intervention in patients with refractory unilateral extremity pain secondary to malignancy. The identification and referral of these patients for treatment requires close collaboration among medical oncologists, neurosurgeons, and pain management specialists, as it is a safe and effective procedure, which can provide an improved quality of life for those suffering from cancer-associated pain.

Further Reading

1. Raslan AM, Cetas JS, McCartney S, Burchiel KJ. Destructive procedures for control of cancer pain: the case for cordotomy. *Journal of Neurosurgery.* 2011;114(1):155–170.
2. Kanpolat Y, Ozdemir M, Al-Beyati E. CT-guided percutaneous cordotomy for intractable pain in what is more than a disease: lung malignancies. *Turkish Neurosurgery.* 2013;23(1):81–87.
3. Gildenberg PL. Ablative spinal cord procedures for cancer pain. In: Andres M, Lozano PLG, Tasker RR, eds. *Textbook of stereotactic and functional neurosurgery* (pp. 2159–2170). Vol 2. Springer 2009.

4. Kanpolat Y. CT-guided percutaneous cervical cordotomy for cancer pain. In: Andres M, Lozano PLG, Tasker RR, eds. *Textbook of stereotactic and functional neurosurgery*. Vol 2. Springer; 2009:2150–2158.
5. Collins KL, Patil PG. Flat-panel fluoroscopy O-arm-guided percutaneous radiofrequency cordotomy: a new technique for the treatment of unilateral cancer pain. *Neurosurgery.* 2013;72(1 Suppl Operative):27–34; discussion 34.
6. Shepherd TM, Hoch MJ, Cohen BA, et al. Palliative CT-guided cordotomy for medically intractable pain in patients with cancer. *American Journal of Neuroradiology.* 2017;38(2):387–390.
7. Raslan AM. Percutaneous computed tomography-guided radiofrequency ablation of upper spinal cord pain pathways for cancer-related pain. *Neurosurgery.* 2008;62(3 Suppl 1):226–233; discussion 233–224.
8. Bain E, Hugel H, Sharma M. Percutaneous cervical cordotomy for the management of pain from cancer: a prospective review of 45 cases. *Journal of Palliative Medicine.* 2013;16(8):901–907.
9. Nagaro T, Adachi N, Tabo E, Kimura S, Arai T, Dote K. New pain following cordotomy: clinical features, mechanisms, and clinical importance. *Journal of Neurosurgery.* 2001;95(3):425–431.
10. Vierck CJ, Jr., Light AR. Effects of combined hemotoxic and anterolateral spinal lesions on nociceptive sensitivity. *Pain.* 1999;83(3):447–457.
11. Kanpolat Y, Ugur HC, Ayten M, Elhan AH. Computed tomography-guided percutaneous cordotomy for intractable pain in malignancy. *Neurosurgery.* 2009;64(3 Suppl):187–193; discussion 193–184.

Spinal Cord Injury Transitional Zone Pain

Oren Sagher

11

Case Presentation

A 55 year-old woman presents with a distant history of American Spinal Injury Association Impairment Score (ASIA) A, T6 spinal cord injury related to a motor vehicle accident. She comes to the clinic, complaining of chest wall pain that began shortly after her injury and that has been progressive since then. The pain is circumferential and is located just above her sensory level. She describes the pain as burning and unremitting. It interferes with her ability to wear clothes, as she finds any skin contact in the painful region extremely unpleasant. She has tried a variety of medications, including narcotics, Neurontin and Elavil, with minimal benefit. An examination confirms complete sensory and motor loss at approximately T6 level, with a band of preserved, but altered sensation that extends rostrally approximately two spinal segments. The patient describes any touch in this region as "numb," but also finds it painful to the touch. Examination of the upper extremities is completely normal.

Questions

1. What is the likely diagnosis?
2. What diagnoses are important to exclude?
3. What is the most appropriate imaging modality?
4. What is the appropriate timing of further workup?

Assessment and Planning

This clinical scenario is classic of a pain syndrome known as Transitional Zone pain, related to the injury and subsequent re-innervation attempt at the level of her prior spinal cord injury. Such pain has distinct neuropathic qualities, and patients commonly describe it a "burning" sensation in a band-like distribution just rostral to the spinal cord injury level. Mechanical allodynia, or the perception of pain in the setting of non-painful stimuli, is also quite common in these cases. The diagnosis is usually a clinical one largely based on the description of the pain, the history of spinal cord injury and the location of symptoms. It is important to exclude any new pathology as an explanation for the pain, such as a developing syrinx, or latent spinal instability. The chief diagnostic imaging modality used in such cases is therefore a spinal MRI. These studies are helpful in delineating the often distorted anatomy of the spinal cord at the level of the prior injury. Any new pathology, such as a spinal cord syrinx, could then be assessed and treated as needed. However, most patients presenting with transitional zone pain do not have evidence of new pathology in the region of the prior injury. In these cases, the clinician must consider treatment modalities that address the presumed mechanism of pain rather than an anatomical lesion.

Oral Boards Review—Diagnostic Pearls

1. Spinal cord transitional zone pain is a clinical diagnosis supported by the history of trauma, the location of symptoms, and their stereotypic nature.
2. Spinal imaging is helpful in excluding incipient instability or a new mass lesion in the spinal canal (such as a syrinx) as causes for the patient's symptoms.
3. On examination, hypesthesia and allodynia, in a band-like distribution directly rostral to the spinal cord injury level, are the hallmarks of this diagnosis.

In the present case, the patient had classic features of transitional zone pain, with the typical band-like area of disordered sensation and pain from roughly T4 to T6 dermatomes. Her CT/myelogram disclosed the expected myelomalacia and arachnoid scarring around T6, with loss of contrast above the level of the injury (Figure 11.1).

Questions

1. How do these clinical and radiological findings influence surgical planning?
2. How would the finding of an expanding spinal cord syrinx affect medical decision making in this case?
3. What would be the potential downsides of surgery targeting the spinal cord above the level of injury?

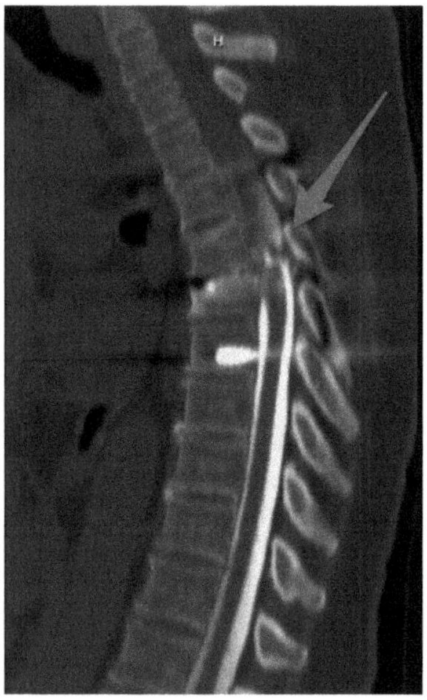

Figure 11.1. Sagittal CT performed after myelography, demonstrating myelomalacia and deformation of the cord in the region of a traumatic spinal cord injury at T6 (arrow). Transitional zone pain is thought to occur just above the region of such traumatic injury.

Decision Making

A history of band-like pain at the junction between normal spinal cord function and absent function related to traumatic spinal cord injury is the *sine-qua-non* of transitional zone pain. In the absence of any developing spinal cord pathology such as a syrinx or spinal instability, the surgical goals are tailored to symptomatic relief. If the pain is intractable to medications such as tricyclic antidepressants or anticonvulsants, surgery is often indicated. The dorsal root entry zone (DREZ) lesion operation, developed by Dr. Blaine Nashold in 1981, was empirically found to have benefit in this condition, and was famously performed on Larry Flynt, the publisher of Hustler Magazine, who suffered from this type of pain after a gunshot wound to the spine. In theory, the origin of this pain relates to aberrant re-innervation of the dorsal horn in the injured spinal cord, causing neuropathic pain in the affected dermatomes. Lesioning of Lissauer's tracts and superficial dorsal horns at these levels, such as that accomplished with a DREZ lesion, presumably destroys these aberrant synapses and therefore treats the pain. Treating such pain with a DREZ lesion does result in "raising" the sensory level to include that band of intermediary sensation, which is expected and should be discussed with the patient. While normally such a new sensory deficit does not result in any functional loss, in specific instances (such as when this loss involves the breast/nipple region) patients may elect to forego this risk.

Surgical Procedure

DREZ lesioning is an open spinal procedure carried out under general anesthetic with a Foley catheter in place, IV access, and invasive arterial blood pressure monitoring. Although it is common to perform DREZ with neuromonitoring when this is done for brachial plexus avulsion pain, patients undergoing DREZ for spinal cord injury transitional zone pain do not have monitorable signals, so this modality is typically not used.

Patients are positioned prone, and spinal levels are identified via X-ray. When the patient has had prior spine surgery, plans should be made to incorporate the rostral segment of the prior surgery in the exposure. A laminectomy is then performed just rostral to the level of injury and typically spans 2 to 3 segments rostrally. The extent of the opening is dictated by the regional anatomy and prior surgical intervention. The dural opening is midline, and often there are extensive arachnoidal adhesions to be lysed once the dura is opened. The dorsal root entry zones are identified bilaterally. Unlike DREZ procedures done for plexus avulsion, the dorsal rootlets are usually preserved in cases done for transitional zone pain. Once the dorsal root entry zones are identified, the lesioning proceeds for the full extent of the planned deafferentation. There are a variety of methods described to accomplish the lesion itself, varying from radiofrequency lesions to laser lesions to lesions accomplished with a microknife. The goal of these lesioning techniques is the same, however—destruction of the superficial layers of the dorsal horn in order to disrupt the aberrant circuits that are the putative source of the pain. In patients undergoing DREZ for transitional zone pain, the lesioning must be performed bilaterally.

Once the lesioning is accomplished, the dura is closed in a watertight fashion, and the incision is closed in layers, in the usual way. Tissue sealants may be used to augment the dural closure, per the surgeon's preference.

Oral Boards Review—Management Pearls

1. Preoperative determination on the location and number of levels to be operated is determined by the location of the spinal cord injury and the extent of the band of pain. Typically, the extent of the DREZ is 2 to 3 levels rostral to the level of injury.
2. It is important to counsel the patient that DREZ would invariably cause numbness in the region of the pain. This is particularly true when the planned DREZ would cause sensory loss around T4, since surgical deafferentation would result in loss of sensation to the nipple.
3. Adequate exposure of the spinal cord bilaterally is important to establish the location of the dorsal root entry zone, especially as the anatomy of the cord may be altered by the nearby injury and scarring.
4. Monitoring of SSEPs and MEPs is not typically helpful, since patients with transitional zone pain usually have a complete spinal cord injury.

Pivot Points

1. Transitional zone pain is difficult to control with neuromodulation, due to the disrupted spinal cord signals at the level of the injury.
2. DREZ lesioning performed in the thoracic location will result in a slightly higher sensory level, but this is usually well tolerated by the patient. Still, this is an important point to counsel patients.
3. DREZ lesioning does not treat pain emanating from completely insensate regions.

Aftercare

Patients are usually observed in an intensive care unit or step down setting on the first night after surgery. They are often kept supine for 2 to 3 days after surgery in order to lessen the risk of cerebrospinal fluid (CSF) egress but are thereafter allowed to resume normal activity.

Complications and Management

The most frequent complication of surgery is CSF leak, due to leakage through the dural incision line. If the CSF is leaking externally, intervention may range from the placement of additional suture reinforcement to contain the leak to insertion of an external lumbar drain to re-exploration of the operative wound with closure of the dural defect. Unplanned neurological deficits related to the procedure are extremely uncommon (excluding the expected sensory loss in the transitional zone). Since these patients have a pre-existing complete neurological injury near the level of the surgery, the risk of additional functional deficit is extremely low.

Oral Boards Review—Complications Pearls

1. A watertight dural closure is extremely important in order to lessen the chance of postoperative CSF leak.
2. The placement of tissue sealants at the time of initial surgery is at the surgeon's discretion, but if a reoperation is performed for CSF leak, these sealants should be incorporated.

Evidence and Outcomes

The evidence supporting the use of DREZ lesioning for transitional zone pain comes predominantly from retrospective case series of this procedure. There is not a great deal of literature documenting success rates, but in general 60 to 70% of patients experience meaningful relief of symptoms with this procedure. Management of transitional zone pain with less invasive means, including medical treatments, blocks, electrical stimulation, or intrathecal medications, has been disappointing.

Further Reading

Awed, A. J., Forbes, J. A., Jermakowicz, W., Eli, I. M., Blumenkopf, B., & Konrad, P. (2013). Experience with 25 years of dorsal root entry zone lesioning at a single institution. *Surgical Neurology International*, *4*(1), 64. http://doi.org/10.4103/2152-7806.112182

Nashold, B. S., & Bullitt, E. (1981). Dorsal root entry zone lesions to control central pain in paraplegics. *Journal of Neurosurgery*, *55*, 414–419.

Siddall, P. J., & Loeser, J. D. (2001). Pain following spinal cord injury. *Spinal Cord*, *39*, 63–73.

Sindou, M. (2011). Surgery in the DREZ for refractory neuropathic pain after spinal cord/cauda equina injury. *World Neurosurgery*, *75*(3-4), 447–448. http://doi.org/10.1016/j.wneu.2011.01.034

Chronic Lumbar Radiculopathy

Spinal Cord Stimulation and Intrathecal Drug Delivery

Brian J. A. Gill, Farhan A. Khan, and Christopher J. Winfree

12

Case Presentation

A 37-year-old woman with type II diabetes mellitus and a long-standing history of low back pain and bilateral leg pain presents for further evaluation. She reports the presence of similar symptoms 2 years earlier. An MRI performed at that time showcased degenerative changes and foraminal stenosis at L5-S1. She subsequently underwent a lumbar decompression and posterior instrumented fusion from L5-S1. Since the surgery she has had persistent axial back and leg pain. She has tried physical therapy and has seen a pain management specialist, who tried to control her pain using various agents, including opioids, antidepressants, anticonvulsants, transcutaneous electrical nerve stimulation (TENS), and interlaminar epidural steroid injections. These treatment regimens have only offered her temporary relief at best. She is now seeing you for further treatment options.

Questions

1. What is the differential diagnosis for this patient's presentation?
2. What are the clinical features of failed back surgery syndrome?
3. What imaging should be obtained for further diagnostic work-up?

Assessment and Planning

This patient likely has failed back surgery syndrome (FBSS), also known as post-laminectomy syndrome. The differential diagnosis for this patient's presentation includes chronic neuropathic pain, FBSS, complex regional pain syndrome, diabetic neuropathy, and ischemic pain secondary to peripheral arterial occlusive disease.

FBSS is characterized by complaints of persistent pain after spine surgery. This pain syndrome may be seen in up to 40% of patients who received a lumbosacral spine surgery for treatment of chronic neuropathic pain.[1] The diagnosis is usually made on the basis of the patient's history and physical examination. Radiographic studies should be obtained in order to rule out the presence of structural causes for the patient's pain syndrome. Upright and flexion-extension lumbar films should be obtained to assess the patient's alignment and to look for evidence of dynamic instability. If the patient has had hardware placed, a non-contrast computed tomography (CT) should be obtained to look for evidence of pseudoarthrosis or fractured instrumentation. Similarly, CT myelography and magnetic resonance imaging (MRI) of the lumbar spine should be obtained to rule out any compression of the neural elements, which would correlate with the patient's presentation.

Oral Boards Review—Diagnostic and Patient Selection Pearls

1. In addition to a thorough history and physical examination, consider the use of a validated pain assessment tool, which may aid in distinguishing the difference between neuropathic and nociceptive back and leg pain.
2. Patients who have structural issues on imaging such as pseudoarthrosis, adjacent level disease, persistent neural element compression, or spinal alignment deformity may be candidates for revision surgery.
3. Patients who are assessed to be good candidates for SCS should receive psychological screening as part of their presurgical evaluation. These tests can identify patients with inadequately controlled psychiatric or psychological disorders who should not be implanted in line with the recommendations from the Neuromodulation Appropriateness Consensus Committee and the USPSTF.[2] While these tests may identify patients who will not respond to SCS, to date there has been no correlation between favorable psychological profile and treatment success.

In the present case, the patient has no neurological deficits on physical examination. Upright and dynamic lumbosacral spine X-rays reveal good position of her previous instrumentation, and good spinal alignment, without evidence of instability (Figure 12.1).

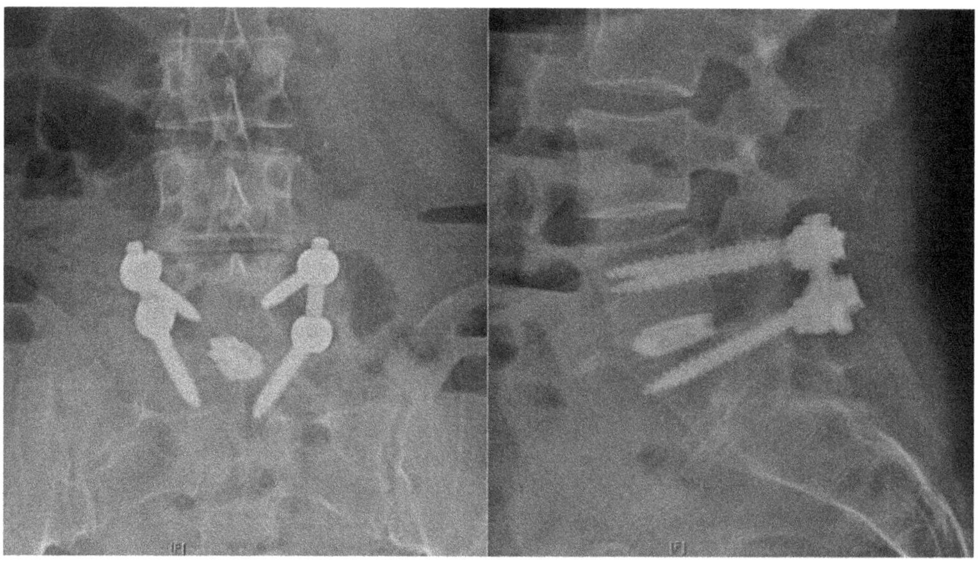

Figure 12.1. Anteroposterior and lateral X-rays demonstrating intact L4-5 hardware without evidence of pseudoarthrosis or instability.

The treating physician notes no clear-cut structural abnormality that would be amenable to surgical decompression on CT myelography or MRI, and the patient has already exhausted a number of reasonable pain management strategies. She could consider a number of additional pain therapies such as opioids and/or medical marijuana as treatment options. The patient, however, has expressed an interest against pursuing more aggressive pharmacotherapy, as she takes care of young children at home.

Questions

1. What are the typical non-surgical management options for patients with chronic neuropathic pain?
2. What are the surgical options for the management of this patient's pain?

Decision Making

Typical pain medication regimens for patients with FBSS usually involve monotherapy with anticonvulsants, antidepressants, baclofen, nonsteroidal anti-inflammatory drugs, or opioids. Failure of monotherapy despite appropriate dose titration is usually followed by combination therapy, also known as multimodal therapy, which may offer better pain relief while allowing the treating physician to lower the doses of the individual agents.

Surgical options for patients with FBSS are typically employed after they have failed appropriate medical management. These options include spinal cord stimulation (SCS), placement of an intrathecal infusion system, or revision lumbar spine surgery. Intrathecal infusion systems allow for the continual administration of analgesic medication in patients refractory to conservative management for neuropathic and nociceptive pain syndromes. Revision lumbar surgery is certainly an option for these patients, particularly in the presence of obvious compressive pathology. In the absence of neurologic deficits, these patients are still candidates for SCS. The decision between the two is a complicated one and depends on the patient's health, as well as the patient's candidacy for longer open procedures.

FBSS is the most common indication for SCS and is ideally suited to patients with greater lower extremity than axial back pain.[2] SCS is a non-ablative and reversible therapy whose effectiveness can be assessed with a 1-week trial using a percutaneous electrode array. The mechanism by which SCS provides analgesia is poorly understood, but probably involves modulation of activity in sensory and pain pathways. The exact mechanism of action likely depends on which waveform is being used, as tonic, high-frequency, and Burst stimulation probably exert somewhat different effects in the spinal cord and more rostral pathways.

Patients who are considered to be good candidates for SCS typically undergo a 1-week trial to assess their response to stimulation. If the patient has sufficient pain relief (commonly considered to be $\geq$ 50%), then they can subsequently undergo permanent implantation. Permanent stimulator systems can either be placed percutaneously or via a laminectomy with a paddle lead. There are a number of different types of spinal cord stimulators in use, each of which has its advantages and disadvantages. There are a variety of electrode sizes and shapes, different waveforms, and rechargeable and non-rechargeable systems. Although clinical trial data support the use of certain types of leads and waveforms in certain clinical situations, the correct choice depends on several factors, including patient preference and physician experience.

The physician elects to proceed with a trial of high-frequency SCS for this case. This has been shown to have a high success rate in the setting of low back and leg pain. An additional advantage of high-frequency stimulation is that there are no discernible paresthesias and thus intraoperative testing is not required.[3,4]

Question

1. What steps can you take to minimize lead migration intraoperatively?

Surgical Procedure

The patient is brought to the operating room and administered general anesthesia with neuromonitoring. She is subsequently placed prone on the operating table and intraoperative fluoroscopy is used to localize her spinal levels. Perioperative intravenous antibiotics are administered. Two large-gauge Tuohy needles are inserted and a paraspinous, loss of resistance technique is used to access the epidural space in the midline. Return of CSF from the Tuohy needle suggests entry into the thecal sac. At this point the needle should be removed. One can attempt entry at a more rostral level if available. CSF will often track along the electrode if the same or a more caudal level is used. This should be avoided. The first electrode is placed in the dorsal epidural space at the top of T8 and the second lead to the midpoint of T9 (Figure 12.2). A lateral fluoroscopic view is obtained to confirm dorsal epidural placement. No intraoperative testing with the patient awake is required with high-frequency stimulation, as it does not produce discernible paresthesias. Intraoperative testing would be required at this

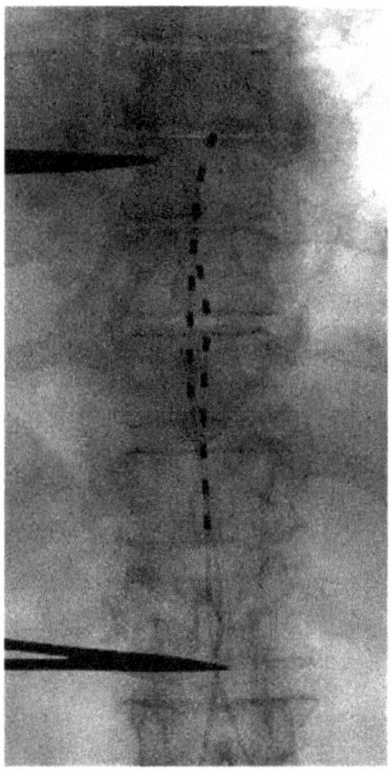

Figure 12.2. Intraoperative anteroposterior fluoroscopic view showing the percutaneous high-frequency SCS array spanning the T8-11 levels. The rostral hemostat is located at the T8-9 interspace while the caudal hemostat is just below the T12 pedicle.

point, however, if a different stimulator system were being used instead. The electrodes are stitched into place and the patient is taken to the post-operative care unit for device programming prior to discharge home.

Oral Boards Review—Operative Management Pearls

1. Stimulation paresthesias (if used) should overlap with the patient's normal pre-operative pain pattern. For patients with low back and leg pain, this best achieved with stimulation of the dorsal columns at the T7-9 spinal levels. Pain below the knee is more reliably treated with electrodes at the T11-L1 levels.[5] High frequency stimulation, as used in this case, utilizes a consistent electrode array, with one electrode advanced to the top of T8 and the second advanced to the midpoint of T9.
2. Needle insertion should occur at least two levels below the target level, if possible. This allows for several centimeters of the lead to lie in the epidural space and decreases the chance electrode migration.

Pivot Points

1. Patients with new or worsening neurological deficits attributable to ongoing neural element compression are not generally candidates for SCS and should be re-evaluated accordingly.
2. The presence of a cardiac electrostimulation devices such as a pacemaker or an automatic implanted cardiac defibrillator does not preclude placement of a SCS system; however, the patient should be cleared by a cardiologist prior to placement.[2]

After Care

Successful trials are defined as at least 50% pain relief while maintaining stable levels of activity in comparison to their preoperative function.[2] At the 1-week postoperative visit, this patient reports only about 25% pain relief, despite multiple reprogramming sessions. The electrodes are removed in the office and other treatment options are discussed. At this point, her options include undergoing another spinal cord stimulator trial with a different waveform or pursuing another form of pain management as outlined earlier in this chapter. The patient chooses to try another form of stimulation and together you decide to try both tonic and Burst stimulation. The former provides stimulation paresthesias, whereas the latter does not.[6]

The second trial is performed with the patient awake in order to place the electrode array in a position, centered at T9, that yields stimulation paresthesias across the patient's low back and legs. The patient reports at the end of the trial that she has 60% pain relief, and she wishes to undergo permanent placement of the device. She is scheduled for permanent placement of a percutaneous system attached to a rechargeable implantable pulse generator.

Complications and Management

The patient returns to her physician's office one year later with complaints of increased low back pain following a minor motor vehicle accident. You recommend that she attempt reprogramming, but this is unsuccessful. The patient additionally reports that the stimulation is no longer in the back, but only the legs. Based on this information, you order imaging to assess whether the electrodes have moved. Plain X-rays show that the electrodes have migrated caudally by spinal two levels, thus explaining the loss of low back coverage.

Given the previous success of SCS in treating her neuropathic pain, it is reasonable to revise her current system. While replacing her current electrodes with the same percutaneous model is an option, her physician elects to place paddle leads at the original lead location (T9) (Figure 12.3) and connect this to her existing implantable pulse generator. In comparison to the percutaneous wire-shaped leads, the paddle leads have a smaller risk of lead migration.[7] Prior to placing paddle leads, an MRI of the thoracic spine should be obtained to ensure that there is sufficient space in the spinal canal to accommodate the paddle lead, as its volume is significantly greater than the percutaneous leads. The procedure is done under general anesthesia and with the aid of neuromonitoring in order to minimize the risk of spinal cord injury.[8]

The patient comes back 18 months later with complaints of incremental loss of response to stimulation. She subsequently undergoes several reprogramming sessions with trials of both tonic and paresthesia-free stimulation but with little effect. She notes that while she can still feel the stimulation in the intended distribution, it no longer relieves her pain. Spinal X-rays show no lead migration or disconnection. At this point, the patient has become a non-responder to multiple spinal cord stimulation waveforms. Given that

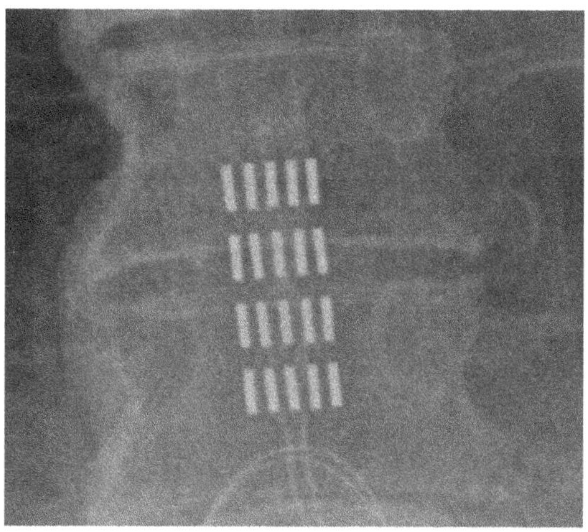

Figure 12.3. Anteroposterior X-ray demonstrating the paddle SCS electrode array spanning the T8-9 levels.

she has failed surgery, physical therapy, exercise, pain management, and neurostimulation, a reasonable option at this point would be to try intrathecal medication.

Historically, intrathecal drug delivery starts with opioids, typically morphine. Chronic intrathecal opioids can be effective at relieving chronic pain but can cause long-term side effects. Given that this patient is in her 30s, one could select a non-opioid alternative for use in her intrathecal system.[9] Based on this, she is offered a trial of intrathecal ziconotide, a synthetic non-opioid analgesic. The trial can be performed either in the operating room or outpatient treatment room. A lumbar puncture is performed, but instead of draining CSF, a dose of ziconotide is injected intrathecally. After an appropriate period of observation, the patient is discharged home. She reports 75% pain relief with the trial, and is offered permanent implantation of a spinal infusion pump system. This is done in the operating room with a general anesthetic and fluoroscopic guidance. The catheter is inserted, in similar fashion to a spinal drain, at a lumbar level and advanced to approximately T12. It is then connected to the programmable pump, which is placed at a subcostal location, centered at but lateral to the level of the umbilicus to avoid contact with the iliac crest and ribcage.

At 1-year follow-up, the patient reports continued pain relief in the 75% range and is happy with her therapy.

Oral Boards Review—Complication Pearls

1. Recurrence of pre-operative pain after a successful period of hardware implantation should raise concern for lead migration. This should be assessed with spinal X-rays. Methods to prevent this include the use of strain relief loops, and ensuring that the nose of the Silastic anchor is pushed through the deep fascia prior to being sutured down.
2. Fever and new onset weakness should raise concern for the development of an epidural abscess. This requires emergent removal of hardware, decompression of the neural elements, and intravenous antibiotics.

Evidence and Outcomes

Evidence for Spinal Cord Stimulation in Neuropathic Pain Syndromes

Prospective clinical trial data suggests that SCS is more effective than revision surgery for patients with FBSS. North et al. performed a randomized controlled trial in which patients with recurrent back and leg pain underwent SCS or revision surgery. In this series, 47% of the patients in the SCS arm and 12% of patients in the repeat surgery arm achieved pain relief levels of at least 50%.[10]

Kumar et al. reported on the results of a multi-center prospective randomized controlled trial comparing SCS and conventional medical management. Patients in the SCS arm reported higher rates of pain relief and improvements in health-related quality of life.[11] Subsequent studies of this patient group have shown that the SCS is more cost-effective than medical management alone.[12,13]

Evidence for Intrathecal Infusion Pumps in Non-malignant Pain Syndromes

Several studies have demonstrated success with using intrathecal infusion pumps for the management of chronic non-cancer-related pain. Wallace et al. reported on the results of a randomized, double-blind, placebo-controlled trial comparing continuous infusions of ziconotide to placebo for patients with chronic non-malignant pain. The ziconotide arm demonstrated greater of pain relief than the placebo arm.[14] Similar success has been demonstrated with opiate infusions.[15]

Further Reading

Deer R, et al. The Polyanalgesic Consensus Conference (PACC): Recommendations on intrathecal drug infusion systems best practices and guidelines. *Neuromodulation*. 2017;20:96.

Deer R, et al. The appropriate use of neurostimulation of the spinal cord and peripheral nervous system for the treatment of chronic pain and ischemic diseases: The Neuromodulation Appropriateness Consensus Committee. *Neuromodulation*. 2014;17:515.

Kapural L, et al. Novel 10-kHz high-frequency therapy (HF10 Therapy) is superior to traditional low-frequency spinal cord stimulation for the treatment of chronic back and leg pain: the SENZA-RCT Randomized Controlled Trial. *Anesthesiology*. 2015;4:851.

Kumar K, et al. Treatment of chronic pain with spinal cord stimulation versus alternative therapies: cost-effectiveness analysis. *Neurosurgery*. 2002;51:106.

Kumar K. et al. Spinal cord stimulation vs. conventional medical management: a prospective, randomized, controlled, multicenter Study of Patients with Failed Back Surgery Syndrome (PROCESS Study). *Neuromodulation*. 2005;8:213.

Levy R, et al. Incidence and avoidance of neurologic complications with paddle type spinal cord stimulation leads. *Neuromodulation*. 2011;14:412.

North R, et al. Spinal cord stimulation electrode design: a prospective, randomized, controlled trial comparing percutaneous with laminectomy electrodes. Part II: clinical outcomes. *Neurosurgery*. 2005;57:990.

North R, et al. Spinal cord stimulation versus reoperation for failed back surgery syndrome: a cost effectiveness and cost utility analysis based on a randomized, controlled trial. *Neurosurgery Online*. 2007;61:361.

References

1. Kumar K, Malik S, Demeria D. Treatment of chronic pain with spinal cord stimulation versus alternative therapies: cost-effectiveness analysis. *Neurosurgery*. Jul 2002;51(1):106–115; discussion 115–106.
2. Deer TR, Mekhail N, Provenzano D, et al. The appropriate use of neurostimulation of the spinal cord and peripheral nervous system for the treatment of chronic pain and ischemic diseases: the Neuromodulation Appropriateness Consensus Committee. *Neuromodulation: Journal of the International Neuromodulation Society*. Aug 2014;17(6):515–550; discussion 550.
3. Kapural L, Yu C, Doust MW, et al. Novel 10-kHz High-frequency therapy (HF10 Therapy) is superior to traditional low-frequency spinal cord stimulation for the treatment of chronic back and leg pain: The SENZA-RCT Randomized Controlled Trial. *Anesthesiology*. Oct 2015;123(4):851–860.

4. Kapural L, Yu C, Doust MW, et al. Comparison of 10-kHz high-frequency and traditional low-frequency spinal cord stimulation for the treatment of chronic back and leg pain: 24-month results from a multicenter, randomized, controlled pivotal trial. *Neurosurgery.* Nov 2016;79(5):667–677.
5. Barolat G, Massaro F, He J, Zeme S, Ketcik B. Mapping of sensory responses to epidural stimulation of the intraspinal neural structures in man. *Journal of Neurosurgery.* Feb 1993;78(2):233–239.
6. Deer T, Slavin KV, Amirdelfan K, et al. Success using neuromodulation with BURST (SUNBURST) study: Results from a prospective, randomized controlled trial using a novel burst waveform. *Neuromodulation: Journal of the International Neuromodulation Society.* Jan 2018;21(1):56–66.
7. North RB, Kidd DH, Petrucci L, Dorsi MJ. Spinal cord stimulation electrode design: a prospective, randomized, controlled trial comparing percutaneous with laminectomy electrodes: part II-clinical outcomes. *Neurosurgery.* Nov 2005;57(5):990–996; discussion 990–996.
8. Levy R, Henderson J, Slavin K, et al. Incidence and avoidance of neurologic complications with paddle type spinal cord stimulation leads. *Neuromodulation: Journal of the International Neuromodulation Society.* Sep-Oct 2011;14(5):412–422; discussion 422.
9. Deer TR, Pope JE, Hayek SM, et al. The Polyanalgesic Consensus Conference (PACC): recommendations on intrathecal drug infusion systems best practices and guidelines. *Neuromodulation: Journal of the International Neuromodulation Society.* Feb 2017;20(2):96–132.
10. North RB, Kidd DH, Farrokhi F, Piantadosi SA. Spinal cord stimulation versus repeated lumbosacral spine surgery for chronic pain: a randomized, controlled trial. *Neurosurgery.* 2005;56(1):98–106; discussion 106–107.
11. Kumar K, North R, Taylor R, et al. Spinal cord stimulation vs. conventional medical management: a prospective, randomized, controlled, multicenter study of patients with failed back surgery syndrome (PROCESS Study). *Neuromodulation: Journal of the International Neuromodulation Society.* Oct 2005;8(4):213–218.
12. Manca A, Kumar K, Taylor RS, et al. Quality of life, resource consumption and costs of spinal cord stimulation versus conventional medical management in neuropathic pain patients with failed back surgery syndrome (PROCESS trial). *European Journal of Pain.* Nov 2008;12(8):1047–1058.
13. Kumar K, Rizvi S. Cost-effectiveness of spinal cord stimulation therapy in management of chronic pain. *Pain Medicine.* Nov 2013;14(11):1631–1649.
14. Wallace MS, Charapata SG, Fisher R, et al. Intrathecal ziconotide in the treatment of chronic nonmalignant pain: a randomized, double-blind, placebo-controlled clinical trial. *Neuromodulation: Journal of the International Neuromodulation Society.* Apr 2006;9(2):75–86.
15. Atli A, Theodore BR, Turk DC, Loeser JD. Intrathecal opioid therapy for chronic nonmalignant pain: a retrospective cohort study with 3-year follow-up. *Pain Medicine.* Jul 2010;11(7):1010–1016.

Intrathecal Drug Therapy for Painful Vertebral Metastases

Sebastian Rubino, Shelby Sabourin, and Julie G. Pilitsis

13

Case Presentation

A 75-year-old woman with a past medical history of coronary artery disease, congestive heart failure, chronic obstructive pulmonary disease, and Crohn's disease with long-term prednisone use presents to the emergency department with increasing lower back pain and unintentional weight loss. She denies any recent trauma and notes the pain is midline. She describes it as, "unbearable to the point where I am unable to walk because the pain is so bad." She denies any weakness, radiculopathies, paresthesias, or difficulties with her bowel or bladder function. On physical exam, she is grossly 5/5 in all muscle groups bilaterally, with normal sensation in all dermatomal distributions. However, she endorses severe tenderness upon direct midline palpation of her lower back.

Questions

1. What is the differential diagnosis? Most likely diagnosis and why?
2. What is the most appropriate imaging modality to help guide treatment strategies?
3. What is the first-line therapy for this diagnosis?

Assessment and Planning

A detailed history and physical exam is the best way to help narrow the list of differential diagnoses. In a patient with unintentional weight loss and no recent trauma, this is most likely an oncologic process. Important questions to help narrow the diagnosis include whether the onset of pain was sudden or progressive, whether the pain is worse in morning or night time, what alleviates and exacerbates the symptoms, and whether the patient is experiencing any bowel, bladder, or sexual dysfunction. Patients with pathologic spine fractures from vertebral metastases typically present with progressive and persistent pain, often increasing in intensity at night.[1] This pain is heightened with sudden movements and typically increases in intensity with time. The physical exam should assess strength, sensation, reflexes, and rectal tone. Patients with osteoporotic lesions, primary bone tumors, or spinal metastases can all have pain to palpation on physical exam. In cases where the pathology causes nerve-root compression or inflammation, radiculopathies and paraspinal muscle spasm may occur.

With regard to diagnostic imaging, plain radiographs may serve as a good screening tool in the outpatient setting, with 73% sensitivity, 100% specificity, and 92% negative predictive value for identifying thoracolumbar fractures.[2] In this patient with severe, immobilizing back pain and concern for an oncologic process given the unintentional weight loss, computed tomography (CT) of the thoracolumbar spine is the most appropriate initial imaging modality, with a sensitivity and specificity of 100% and 97%, respectively.[2] As in this case, it is important to order a CT of the chest, abdomen, and pelvis with and without contrast as part of the metastatic work-up and to simultaneously evaluate the spine. Unfortunately, the scan in this patient was positive for a right upper lobe spiculated mass measuring 3.2 × 3.2 × 3.6 cm abutting the superior mediastinum by approximately 1.8 cm without discernible encasement of the adjacent vessels, concerning for primary lung cancer. The thoracolumbar spine was positive for numerous compression fractures from the T11 through L5 level with associated neuroforaminal stenosis. In order to better assess for canal compromise, MRI with and without gadolinium should be obtained next. The MRI in this patient revealed the previously identified compression fractures without any major compression of the thecal sac (Figure 13.1A). Unfortunately, the patient was unable to tolerate gadolinium administration secondary to a prior allergic reaction. Given the patient's history, physical exam, and imaging findings, the most likely diagnosis is pathologic compression fractures secondary to her metastatic lung cancer.

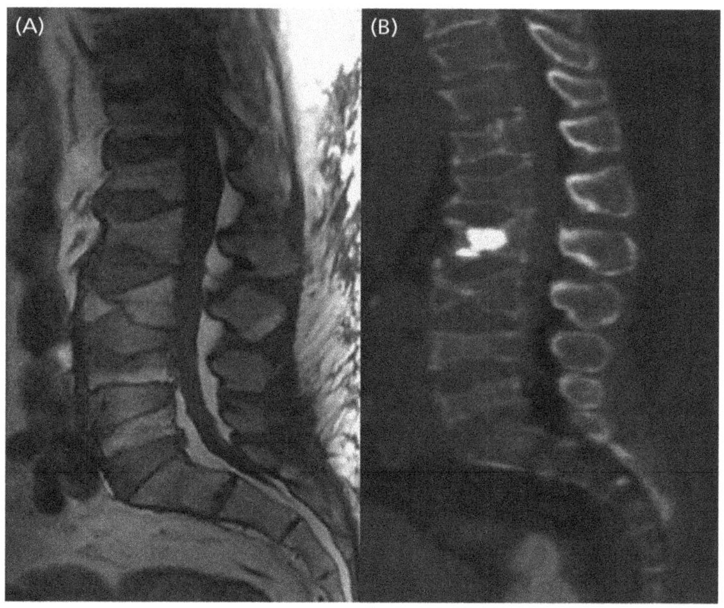

Figure 13.1. A. Magnetic resonance imaging T1 sequence illustrating contiguous compression fractures from T11 to L5 without major compression of the thecal sac. B. Lumbar computed tomography with sagittal reconstruction illustrating the multiple compression fractures and L2 vertebral body opacification of methyl methacrylate after L2 kyphoplasty.

Oral Boards Review—Diagnostic Pearls

1. Differentiating between vertebral metastases and osteoporotic lesions can be difficult. History, physical exam, and imaging findings must be integrated in order to make the correct diagnosis.
2. Plain radiographs may serve as a good screening tool in the outpatient setting but computed tomography of the spine is the most appropriate initial diagnostic test in the hospital setting.
3. Flexion and extension radiographs are also useful in assessing spinal stability.
4. MRI with and without contrast is also needed to determine full extent of oncologic burden and degree of canal compromise.

Medical management is the first line of treatment for pain control in patients with painful vertebral metastases. First-line agents include paracetamol, non-steroidal anti-inflammatory drugs (NSAIDs), neuropathic pain agents, bisphosphonates, and opioids. Maximal dosing strategies include paracetamol (4000mg/day), ibuprofen (2400 mg/day), naproxen (1000 mg/day), diclofenac (200 mg/day), pregabalin (600 mg/day), and gabapentin (3600 mg/day).[3] Both oral and intravenous bisphosphonates may be used in the treatment of secondary osteoporosis from malignancy; some examples include alendronate (70 mg/week), risedronate (35 mg/week), or ibandronate sodium (150 mg/month).[4] As recommended by the Centers for Disease Control, opioid dosing should remain below 90 morphine milligram equivalents per day.[5] Furthermore, pain associated with pathologic fractures is often a result of spinal instability and treatment of the instability should occur concomitantly with medical management. Specific treatments for spinal instability depend on the patient's overall prognosis and comorbidities, but some options may include resection of the tumor with spinal reconstruction, radiation therapy, and vertebroplasty or kyphoplasty.[6] Surgery, chemotherapy, and radiation therapy aim to decrease tumor burden, provide structural support, as well as limit motion over the involved vertebral segment.

Our patient underwent a video-assisted thoracoscopic surgery for biopsy of her lung mass and the pathology confirmed non-small cell lung carcinoma. She was initially placed on paracetamol, ibuprofen, gabapentin, and oxycodone to help with her lower back pain. This regimen only provided brief, non-sustained relief. Oxycontin was also added in attempts to provide more continuous pain control. The combined regimen was limited by somnolence, respiratory depression, and lack of adequate pain control. The patient subsequently was scheduled to undergo multi-level lumbar kyphoplasty, but was only able to receive an L2 kyphoplasty secondary to her large body habitus (Figure 13.1B). This intervention also did not provide any significant level of pain relief.

Questions

1. What surgical interventions can be offered to patients with pain from vertebral metastases?
2. What is the proposed mechanism of action of these interventions?

Decision Making

For patients in whom traditional medical management has failed or in whom oncologic burden or commodities are too great to under any significant stabilization procedures, intrathecal drug therapy (IDT) can serve as an effective adjunct to improve pain control, mobility, and quality of life. Common analgesics administered intrathecally include FDA approved morphine (0.1–0.5 mg/day) and ziconotide (0.5-–2.4 μg/day), while bupivacaine (1–4 mg/day), hydromorphone (0.02–0.50 mg/day), and clonidine (40–100 μg/day) may also be used off label.[7] Selection of the treatment dose for IDT is based on the Morphine Equivalent Dose the patient is receiving orally or intravenously and a trial of the IDT should be performed prior to proceeding to permanent implantation. The trial offers an opportunity to help determine which medication and dose may most effectively relieve the patient's pain.

A patient with a prior history of cancer who develops vertebral metastases is often faced with multiple treatment options. Although radiation therapy, primary surgery, and kyphoplasty have shown high efficacy in clinical trials[6] and primarily seek to address oncologic burden and structural instability, morbidity from these procedures can decrease the quality of life for a significant portion of a patient's remaining lifespan. IDT delivery systems allow patients to receive lower dosages of analgesics, with a lower incidence of side effects, and lead to an improved quality of life.[8] These systems afford patients pain relief, while preserving cognizance that would otherwise be affected with high levels of systemic opioids, and enable patients to spend more time at home rather than in a hospital or hospice setting. Implanted intrathecal pumps can provide either nociceptive or neuropathic pain relief, depending on the medication administered, with minimal maintenance and programming.

Questions

1. In what anatomical location do you place the intrathecal catheter when treating vertebral metastases?
2. Where do most catheters get kinked during implant surgery?

Surgical Procedure

Intrathecal Pump Implantation

Implantation of intrathecal drug pumps is performed using a c-arm for fluoroscopic guidance. Before operating, the patient is positioned in the lateral decubitus position on top of a bean bag such that the side where the pump will be placed is facing upward. We identify and mark the locations of the L3-4 and T7-8 interspaces using fluoroscopy; a radiopaque EKG lead is placed at the T7-8 interspace so that we can identify the level under fluoroscopy once the sterile drapes are applied (Figure 13.2). The L3-4 interspace marks the entry point of our catheter needle, while the T7-8 interspace is the final level where the distal tip of the catheter must reach. At this point, a midline incision is made over the L3-4 interspace such that the lumbar fascia can be exposed. Using c-arm fluoroscopy for guidance, a lumbar puncture is performed with the catheter needle at a 30° cephalad angulation, and the catheter is threaded to approximately the T7-8 interspace. Most catheters get kinked upon entry into the thecal sac if the angle is too obtuse. If

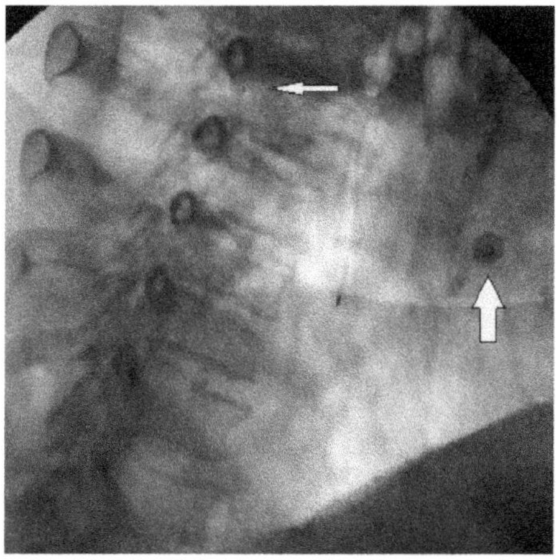

Figure 13.2. Intraoperative x-ray confirmation of the intrathecal catheter reaching the T7 level (thin arrow) using the pre-operatively placed EKG lead (thick arrow) as a reference point for the T7-8 interspace.

there is difficulty accessing the intrathecal sac via the L3-4 interspace with proper angulation, the incision may be extended in the cephalad direction so the needle may enter via the L2-3 interspace. We typically use 2-0 silk sutures to secure an anchor around the catheter to the fascia once the correct location is confirmed with fluoroscopy. We next place additional silk sutures to ensure the anchor is flush with the fascia. A small strain relief loop is made and the area is checked to ensure there are no kinks. An abdominal pocket is then created for the pump by making an incision at the desired location midway between the lowest rib and the anterior iliac spine. The fascia of the external oblique muscle is exposed and an approximately 4-inch by 5-inch subcutaneous pocket is created using Bovie electrocautery and gentle blunt dissection. We subsequently pass the catheter from the lumbar incision to the abdominal incision using a shunt passer. The catheter is connected to the pump, cerebrospinal fluid is aspirated through the pump to ensure catheter patency, and the pump is placed in the pocket and sutured to the fascia. At this point, we irrigate the pocket and lumbar incision with bacitracin-containing irrigation solution, place vancomycin powder in both incisions, and close using 3-0 vicryl sutures and staples. Once placement of the pump is complete, we activate the device and initiate intrathecal saline therapy.

Post-operative Programming

Following surgery, the pump will need to be filled with the appropriate medication and programmed to fit the needs of the individual. Although there is no one formula that has proven effective in converting pre-operative oral medications to intrathecal dosages, programming typically begins with a dose of 0.1–0.5 mg of morphine equivalents per day and is increased gradually to reach the targeted dosage. The appropriate target dosage is the lowest dose during programming that relieves pain with minimal or no harmful side effects. If patients are weaned off systemic opioids prior to undergoing pump implantation, intrathecal analgesics should be micro-dosed during the initial infusion titration to avoid overdose.

Oral Boards Review—Management Pearls

1. In order to correctly place the catheter at your pre-planned level, use c-arm fluoroscopy to obtain a lateral x-ray (anteroposterior to the laterally positioned patient) and mark the level with an EKG lead; simultaneously mark your entry level and plan your lumbar incision. This enables you to have a guiding landmark after the sterile drapes are applied.
2. The catheter must extend a minimum of 3 vertebral bodies above the entry point to be considered stable.
3. It is important to aspirate cerebrospinal fluid from the pump once the catheter is connected to confirm catheter patency.

Pivot Points

1. Care should be taken when placing intrathecal catheters in patients with cord compression and should be timed in coordination with radiation therapy and surgery where indicated.
2. Intrathecal catheters for IDT delivery systems may be placed at time of decompressive or reconstructive surgery if the patient has considerable pain that is not expected to meaningfully improve following resection or stabilization.
3. Laminectomy for open catheter placement may be needed for patients with previous lumbar surgeries or aberrant anatomy preventing percutaneous access to the thecal sac.
4. Intraoperative neuromonitoring may be used to mitigate the risks associated with difficult percutaneous access.

Aftercare

Patients are admitted overnight for neurological monitoring. We ask them to remain flat, although they may roll side to side with one pillow until the next morning to prevent cerebrospinal fluid headache. Patients should be carefully monitored to determine if the dose is too high (somnolence) or too low (continued severe pain). Oral and intravenous medications must be carefully dosed in consideration with the initial infusion of IDT pain medications. We place the patients in an abdominal binder for two weeks as tolerated and obtain x-rays to use as comparison over time or to help access the device in the future.

Complications and Management

Some complications of IDT are similar to those of systemic opioid use such as constipation, nausea, pruritus, urinary retention, hypotension, opioid-induced hyperanalgesia, hypogonadotropic hypogonadism, immunologic compromise, headaches, and respiratory depression.[9] Other complications include formation of intrathecal granulomas, seromas, hygromas, and bacterial meningitis.[10] Patients with constipation, nausea, and pruritus may take over-the-counter medications for symptomatic relief. The cardiovascular, endocrine, immune, respiratory, and hyperanalgesia complications may improve with dose reduction, drug rotation, and removal of intrathecal opioids.[7] The incidence of intrathecal granulomas is between approximately 0.5% and 3%.[11] Diagnosis based on clinical suspicion can be made with a T1 contrasted MRI or CT myelogram. Mild symptoms can be managed by stopping the infusion or replacing the drug with sterile saline for infusion. However, if causing neurological deficits, the pump and catheter should be removed to avoid the risk of permanent paralysis.

Oral Boards Review—Complications Pearls

1. Careful preoperative assessment and optimization will help minimize complications.
2. If a patient's pain is too severe to return home, IDT should be aggressively adjusted with great care to balance total morphine equivalent dosing safely.
3. IDT doses are often very high and if there is a malfunction, patients may go into withdrawal, which is life threatening and must be treated immediately. Signs and symptoms of IDT withdrawal include high fevers, tachypnea, tachycardia, and return of severe pain.
4. Granulomas have been reported with high morphine IDT dosages.

Evidence and Outcomes

Intrathecal delivery of morphine in human subjects with severe, intractable oncologic pain was first reported by Wang et al. in 1978.[12] More recent studies, including a prospective open-label study by Rauck et al., found that greater than 80% of patients with implantation of intrathecal drug delivery systems had 50% or greater reduction in cancer pain at up to 4-month follow-up.[13] A 2016 prospective cohort study in patients with advanced malignancies and mean follow-up of 6.97 months found that 52.3% of patients with intrathecal drug delivery systems had 50% or greater pain relief up to 1 week before their death.[14] Lastly, a 2018 retrospective study by Sayed et al. found that the median pain score—on a scale from 0 to 10—decreased by 3.2 points in patients with severe cancer pain and intrathecal pain pump implantation.[15] As indicated by these studies and others, IDT is a safe and effective adjunct to the treatment of intractable oncologic pain in patients who have failed conservative medical management and are unwilling or unable to undergo larger surgical procedures.

Further Reading

1. Kienstra GE, Terwee CB, Dekker FW, et al. Prediction of spinal epidural metastases. *Arch Neurol.* 2000;57(5):690–695.
2. Berry GE, Adams S, Harris MB, et al. Are plain radiographs of the spine necessary during evaluation after blunt trauma? Accuracy of screening torso computed tomography in thoracic/lumbar spine fracture diagnosis. *J Trauma.* 2005;59(6):1410–1413; discussion 1413.

3. Ripamonti CI, Bandieri E, Roila F, Group EGW. Management of cancer pain: ESMO Clinical Practice Guidelines. *Ann Oncol.* 2011;22 Suppl 6:vi 69–77.
4. Hofbauer LC, Hamann C, Ebeling PR. Approach to the patient with secondary osteoporosis. *Eur J Endocrinol.* 2010;162(6):1009–1020.
5. Dowell D, Haegerich TM, Chou R. CDC Guideline for Prescribing Opioids for Chronic Pain—United States, 2016. *JAMA.* 2016;315(15):1624–1645.
6. Lutz S. The role of radiation therapy in controlling painful bone metastases. *Curr Pain Headache Rep.* 2012;16(4):300–306.
7. Shah R, Baqai-Stern A, Gulati A. Managing intrathecal drug delivery (ITDD) in cancer patients. *Curr Pain Headache Rep.* 2015;19(6):20.
8. De Andres J, Asensio-Samper JM, Fabregat-Cid G. Intrathecal delivery of analgesics. *Methods Mol Biol.* 2014;1141:249–278.
9. Gulati A, Puttanniah V, Hung J, Malhotra V. Considerations for evaluating the use of intrathecal drug delivery in the oncologic patient. *Curr Pain Headache Rep.* 2014;18(2):391.
10. Czernicki M, Sinovich G, Mihaylov I, et al. Intrathecal drug delivery for chronic pain management-scope, limitations and future. *J Clin Monit Comput.* 2015;29(2):241–249.
11. Deer TR. A prospective analysis of intrathecal granuloma in chronic pain patients: a review of the literature and report of a surveillance study. *Pain Physician.* 2004;7(2):225–228.
12. Wang JK, Nauss LA, Thomas JE. Pain relief by intrathecally applied morphine in man. *Anesthesiology.* 1979;50(2):149–151.
13. Rauck RL, Cherry D, Boyer MF, Kosek P, Dunn J, Alo K. Long-term intrathecal opioid therapy with a patient-activated, implanted delivery system for the treatment of refractory cancer pain. *J Pain.* 2003;4(8):441–447.
14. Zheng S, He L, Yang X, Li X, Yang Z. Evaluation of intrathecal drug delivery system for intractable pain in advanced malignancies: A prospective cohort study. *Medicine (Baltimore).* 2017;96(11):e6354.
15. Sayed D, Monroe F, Orr WN, et al. Retrospective analysis of intrathecal drug delivery: outcomes, efficacy, and risk for cancer-related pain at a high volume academic medical center. *Neuromodulation.* 2018.

Pelvic/Visceral Cancer Pain

Ashwin Viswanathan

14

Case Presentation

A 64-year-old woman with a history of hepatic epithelioid hemangioendothelioma presents with persistent abdominal pain. The pain is located in the epigastric region, as well as the right upper quadrant of the abdomen. She is in pain constantly, and there is no increased pain to palpation. She has no other sites of pain.

The patient has been seen by the Pain Medicine service and was first optimized on opioids up to a morphine equivalent daily dosage of 150 mg. Despite opioid intake, she has had persistent pain. The patient also underwent a splanchnic nerve block and splanchnic neurolysis with only transient improvement in her symptoms. She is referred for further treatment options for her cancer-related pain.

Questions

1. What type of pain does this patient have?
2. How is pain transmitted in the spinal cord?
3. What are the interventional options for treating her pain?

Assessment and Planning

This patient is presenting with symptoms attributable to visceral cancer pain. Although somatic pain is transmitted in the anterolateral spinothalamic tract, visceral pain travels in an alternate pain pathway—the postsynaptic dorsal columns visceral pain pathway. This pain pathway ascends along the medial border of the dorsal columns. Animal studies in both rodents and primates have supported the presence of this pathway, and surgical experience in humans has documented effective relief of visceral pain when this pathway is sectioned.

As this patient has been optimized on oral opioids and has undergone percutaneous neurolysis without long-term benefit, surgical options should be considered. There are two principal means through which visceral pain can be treated. First, intrathecal opioids are a commonly used therapy for the management of refractory visceral cancer pain. The ideal candidate for intrathecal opioids is the patient who experiences pain relief with opioids but has intolerable systemic side effects such as lethargy or confusion with opioid administration. Patients deemed appropriate candidates for intrathecal therapy may benefit from undergoing a trial of intrathecal opioids via lumbar puncture.

Questions

1. What are two surgical options for visceral cancer pain?
2. What therapy can be used in patients that have relief but side effects with systemic opioids?
3. What fibers does midline myelotomy seek to disrupt?

Oral Boards Review—Diagnostic Pearls

1. Validated patient reported outcomes such as the Edmonton Symptom Assessment Scale and the Brief Pain Inventory are essential in quantifying symptom burden pre- and postoperatively.
2. Collaboration with oncologists, pain medicine physicians, and palliative care physicians can ensure that patients have been aggressively treated with both pharmacological and non-pharmacological pain treatments prior to surgical intervention.
3. Nerve blocks (splanchnic, celiac, and hypogastric) can help identify the source of the pain and can be useful in differentiating somatic from visceral pain.

The second surgical consideration for patients with intractable visceral pain is midline myelotomy. The first surgical myelotomies sought to interrupt the commissural fibers of the spinothalamic tract. However, it was noted that patients had more widespread pain relief than would be expected from only interrupting the decussating pathways. Hence both clinical and basic science experience lead to the recognition of a visceral pain pathway, which ascends in between the dorsal columns. More recent approaches to myelotomy have focused on interrupting this ascending pathway rather than the commissural fibers of the spinothalamic tract.

Questions

1. What are the advantages of intrathecal opioids in the management of refractory cancer pain?
2. What is the difference between a commissural myelotomy and a punctate midline myelotomy?
3. What are three techniques for performing a punctate midline myelotomy?

Decision Making

Both intrathecal drug delivery and midline myelotomy are appropriate options to offer this patient. The advantages and limitations of both approaches should be discussed in detail with the patient.

The principal advantage of intrathecal drug delivery is that it is a very low-risk intervention. There is a 1% risk of infection and catheter malfunction with this procedure. However, there are two downsides of this approach. First, intrathecal drug delivery requires routine maintenance with pump refills every 3 months. Second, if the patient was not getting some relief of pain with oral opioids, there is a risk that she will not get relief of pain with intrathecal opioids as well.

One main advantage of midline myelotomy is that it is a one-time intervention that can bring dramatic and immediate pain relief to the patient with no further follow-up needed for her pain. The disadvantage of myelotomy is that it is a surgical procedure on the spinal cord and carries the risk of injuring both the dorsal columns and the corticospinal tract. In addition, myelotomy performed via laminectomy carries the additional risk of general anesthesia and cerebrospinal fluid (CSF) leak due to opening the dura.

Percutaneous approaches to perform midline myelotomy can also be considered. A radiofrequency technique at the occipito-cervical level is well tolerated in the advanced cancer patient who may have contraindications to surgery under general anesthesia or laminectomy. A percutaneous mechanical myelotomy has also been described more than once in the literature, in which a spinal angiocatheter is inserted into the midline of the thoracic spinal cord to the antero-posterior midpoint of the spinal cord. The needle position and trajectory for both percutaneous approaches are confirmed using real-time CT guidance.

For the radiofrequency approach, a 26 G radiofrequency electrode of diameter 0.46 mm can be used. This is slightly larger than the standard cordotomy electrode and has been reported to have more durable outcomes as compared with a smaller electrode. The percutaneous approach is favored in patients with thrombocytopenia, patients on chemotherapy, and in patients for whom a spine operation may be too disruptive with end-of-life goals.

Surgical Procedure

Open, punctate midline myelotomy is performed in the prone position under general anesthesia. The level for the myelotomy is selected based on the location of the patient's pain. For patients with upper abdominal pain, a lesion is placed at the T3 level. For patients with perineal pain, a lesion is made at the T6 level. The goal is to interrupt the ascending visceral pain pathway rostral to the source of pain.

Once the level is confirmed using AP fluoroscopy, a one or one-and–a-half level laminectomy is performed. The laminectomy is carried out widely enough to allow visualization of root entry zones bilaterally. Prior to dural opening, meticulous hemostasis is achieved. The dura is opened in the midline, and dural retention sutures are placed bilaterally. Small hemoclips may be useful to keep the pia out of the region of interest. The midline is identified by determining the midpoint of the root entry zones and by visualizing the point where the penetrating arterioles enter the dorsal medial sulcus. Attempt should be made to preserve a dorsal median vein, although sacrifice of this vein can be performed if needed.

Once the midline has been carefully identified, microbipolars are used to coagulate the proposed location for the myelotomy. A 16-gauge angiocatheter is a useful tool for creating the mechanical lesion in the spinal cord. The catheter portion of the angiocatheter can be cut to expose a 5 mm exposed tip. The goal of myelotomy is to create a lesion that extends 0.5 mm bilaterally and which extends 5 mm in depth. This should be an adequate depth to reach the central canal of the spinal cord.

Once the lesion is created, meticulous hemostasis is achieved using Gelgoam and the judicious use of bipolar cautery. Running 4-0 silk suture is used to close the dura in a watertight manner. A thorough fascial closure is also essential for preventing postoperative cerebrospinal fluid leaks.

For percutaneous CT-guided techniques, lumbar puncture with instillation of contrast into the lumbar cistern will aid in visualization of the spinal cord and placement of the spinal needle. The patient is positioned in the prone position ideally. For patients who cannot tolerate the prone position due to abdominal pain, the lateral position can also be used. The critical technical detail is to ensure that the spinal needle and hence radiofrequency (RF) electrode is in the midline of the spinal cord. Once the RF electrode is placed, motor stimulation can be used at 2 Hz to ensure a safe distance from the corticospinal tract. The RF electrode is placed in the anteroposterior midpoint of the spinal cord where an RF ablation is performed at 75–80 C for 60 seconds. The RF electrode is withdrawn 2 mm and a second RF ablation is performed to lesion the anterior-posterior extent of the dorsal columns visceral pain pathway.

Oral Boards Review—Management Pearls

1. Intrathecal opioids have been shown in a randomized controlled study to reduce the toxicity associated with systemic opioid administration.
2. Intraoperative neurophysiological monitoring (motor and sensory) should be used during punctate midline myelotomy to minimize surgical complications.
3. Stimulation of the dorsal columns while recording somatosensory evoked potentials from scalp electrodes can help in identifying the physiological midline of the spinal cord.

Aftercare

Postoperatively, the patient is admitted for observation and pain control. A careful neurological exam is performed to assess for interruption in dorsal columns function and to assess for a change in motor strength due to injury of the corticospinal tract. The patient is mobilized as soon as feasible, with no period of bedrest. Within 24 to 48 hours post-procedure, the patient should experience an improvement in their visceral pain. Opioids can be reduced in conjuncture with the patient's oncologist or pain physician.

Pivot Points

1. Should the patient not receive benefit from myelotomy, post-procedure MRI can be used to quantify the spinal cord lesion.
2. Intrathecal therapy can be used in conjunction with neuroablation for patients with highly refractory pain syndromes.
3. For patients who fail to improve after percutaneous radiofrequency myelotomy, consideration can still be given to open punctate myelotomy, under the rationale that the RF lesion may not have been adequate in size.

Complications and Management

Myelotomy is generally a safe procedure, and risks associated with myelotomy are often acceptable for the patient suffering from intractable cancer pain. Up to 25% of patients may experience symptoms attributable to interruption of the dorsal columns. This can lead to tingling of the feet and altered proprioception.

The incidence of motor weakness following puncture myelotomy is low. Based on published experience, there is a less than a 5% incidence of motor deficit or change in bowel or bladder patterns after myelotomy.

Other surgical complications include CSF leak through the skin. Should a patient experience CSF leak, attempts can be made to oversew the incision with the use of a surgical adhesive. However, a low threshold should exist for returning the patient to the OR for identification of the leak site and proper primary closure.

Oral Boards Review—Complications Pearls

1. Careful attention to dural and fascial closure is essential to avoid postoperative CSF leak.
2. The lesion depth for punctate myelotomy should be no more than 5 mm to avoid injury to the anterior spinal artery.
3. For patients undergoing active chemotherapy, percutaneous approaches are preferred as they carry minimal to no risk of CSF leak or puncture site infection.

Evidence and Outcomes

At least 9 series have been reported in the literature, representing more than 110 patients who have undergone punctate midline myelotomy. The largest series by Schvarcz was published in 1976 and reported that 84% of 45 patients had a satisfactory outcome. However, as with outcome studies for many neuroablative procedures, conclusions as to the efficacy of myelotomy are limited by short survival postoperatively due to malignancy and very heterogeneous outcome metrics used.

In 1984, Gildenberg et al. reported good outcomes in 9 of 12 patients undergoing open limited myelotomy, and in 2000, Nauta reported that 5 out of 6 patients experienced greater than a 30% reduction in pain intensity. Our center has had better pain outcomes when using an open surgical technique for myelotomy as compared with a percutaneous approach. Hence, we preferentially use an open technique if the patient can tolerate it. In patients who cannot tolerate an open surgery, a percutaneous radiofrequency myelotomy is offered targeting the dorsal columns visceral pain pathway at the occipiut-C1 level.

Further Reading

Gildenberg PL, Hirshberg RM. Limited myelotomy for the treatment of intractable cancer pain. J Neurol Neurosurg Psychiatry. Jan 1984;47(1):94–96.

Kanpolat Y, Savas A, Caglar S, Akyar S. Computerized tomography-guided percutaneous extralemniscal myelotomy. Neurosurg Focus. Jan 15 1997;2(1):e5.

Nauta HJ, Hewitt E, Westlund KN, Willis WD, Jr. Surgical interruption of a midline dorsal column visceral pain pathway. Case report and review of the literature. J Neurosurg. Mar 1997;86(3):538–542.

Nauta HJ, Soukup VM, Fabian RH, et al. Punctate midline myelotomy for the relief of visceral cancer pain. J Neurosurg. Apr 2000;92(2 Suppl):125–130.

Vedantam A, Koyyalagunta D, Bruel BM, Dougherty PM, Viswanathan A. Limited midline myelotomy for intractable visceral pain: surgical techniques and outcomes. Neurosurgery. 2018;83(4):783–789.

Viswanathan A, Burton AW, Rekito A, McCutcheon IE. Commissural myelotomy in the treatment of intractable visceral pain: technique and outcomes. Stereotact Funct Neurosurg. 2010;88(6):374–382.

Willis WD, Al-Chaer ED, Quast MJ, Westlund KN. A visceral pain pathway in the dorsal column of the spinal cord. Proc Natl Acad Sci USA. 1999 Jul 6;96(14):7675–7679.

Painful Diabetic Neuropathy

Emily Lehmann Levin

15

Case Presentation

A 68-year-old man with a 15-year history of type II diabetes mellitus has had complaints of numbness and burning pain in bilateral feet, which has been progressive over the last 5 years. It initially started in his toes, but has spread to involve feet in a stocking distribution. The feet feel numb, with pins and needles, but at the same time a light touch is exquisitely painful. On exam, he has full strength in all four extremities. He reports decreased sensation to light touch in a stocking distribution in his feet up to the ankles. He has decreased proprioception at the great toes. His primary care provider has managed with gabapentin initially, followed by pregabalin. He is also on amitriptyline for depression, and these have had little effect on his foot pain. The patient wishes to avoid opioids. The allodynia is interfering with sleep and is causing significant distress.

Questions

1. What is the likely diagnosis?
2. What diagnoses are important to exclude?
3. What further testing is most appropriate?
4. What is the appropriate treatment algorithm?

Assessment and Planning

The neurosurgeon suspects that this patient has painful neuropathy, likely secondary to chronic diabetes, due to the symmetric, distal distribution, and predominantly nocturnal symptoms. There was no significant history of alcohol abuse or heavy metal exposure, and no evidence of B12 deficiency. Nerve conduction study was performed and was consistent with small fiber distal, symmetric polyneuropathy.

Questions

1. How does one choose a treatment for painful diabetic neuropathy?
2. When is surgical treatment appropriate?

Decision Making

Initial management of painful diabetic neuropathy is non-surgical. Improved glucose control with goal hemoglobin A1C of 6–7% is important. Pharmacologic management is with tricyclic antidepressants, serotonin and norepinephrine reuptake inhibitors, and anti-epileptics, predominantly gabapentin and pregabalin. Surgical treatment is reserved for those patients with severe symptoms, with significantly impaired quality of life, for whom medications have not provided significant relief, as in the patient described in this case. It should be noted, however, that patients with dense numbness associated with their neuropathy tend to respond poorly to spinal cord stimulation. In this individual, a trial of spinal cord stimulation was recommended.

Surgical Procedure

Placement of epidural stimulation electrodes may be accomplished in a number of ways. In the simplest technique, the electrode may be placed percutaneously through a Tuohy needle, with the leads connected to a generator that may be either external (temporary) or implanted. At the other end of the range, a single-level laminotomy may be performed for placement of a paddle-style electrode. The percutaneous lead has the advantage of being able to be advanced over a number of spinal segments, allowing easier adjustment of the stimulated level to optimize symptom control. There is less tissue disturbance associated with the percutaneous lead, when compared to the paddle-style electrode. However, bilateral stimulation often requires the placement of two percutaneous leads. In addition, the broad footprint of the paddle-shaped electrode provides it with greater stability and durability, and is less associated with lead migration and damage. For the purposes of this chapter, we will focus on paddle-lead placement.

These procedures are traditionally performed in a conscious patient, using local anesthetics and mild sedation to allow the patient to assist in optimal placement of the stimulating electrode.

A trial of stimulation prior to permanent implantation is typically performed to ensure that the spinal cord stimulation provides significant pain relief. This involves an initial lead placement with connection to an external generator, allowing for evaluation of the treatment for several days. The electrodes may then be used permanently or changed at the time of generator implantation.

Determination of the spinal level for electrode insertion and placement is key to successful stimulation. The location of pain treated and the type of electrode being placed guide the level of insertion. Paddle-type electrodes may generally only be placed one to two levels cranial to the location of the laminotomy. The target level for the electrical contacts varies by patient and pain region being treated. Common target levels for lower extremity coverage range from T8 to T12, spanning the lumbar enlargement of the spinal cord. For distal coverage, i.e. foot pain, the typical stimulation level is closer to T12 (see Figure 15.1).

The paddle electrode is placed with the patient in the prone position. A fluoroscope is positioned antero-posterior and the vertebral level is identified. Following generous administration of local anesthetic, a midline incision is made over the interspace through which the electrode will be placed. The paraspinous muscles are cleared from the spinous processes and lamina bilaterally, the inferior portion of the cranial lamina is resected, and the ligamentum flavum is carefully removed. The epidural space is explored cranially to ensure that there are no adhesions and the electrode is placed under visual

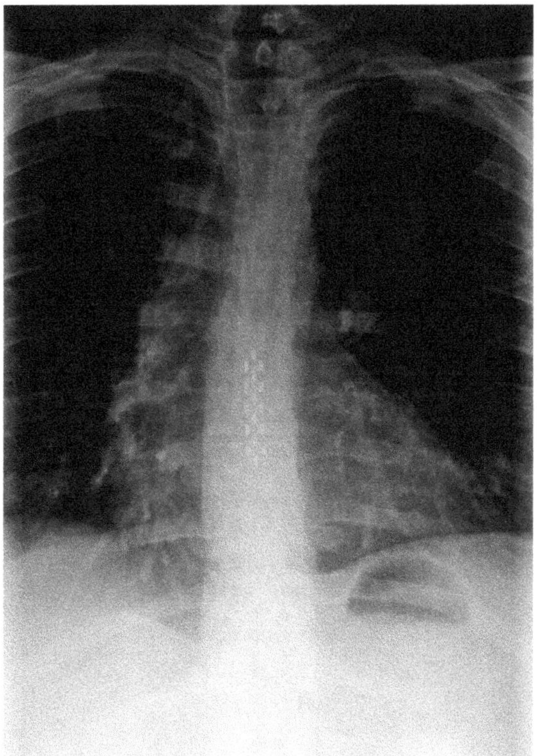

Figure 15.1. AP radiograph demonstrating a paddle-type spinal cord stimulator lead in the epidural space centered at the T8-9 level.

and AP fluoroscopic guidance. With the advent of minimally invasive spine surgery techniques, some have advocated their use to decrease post-operative surgical pain and recovery time.

Often at this point, a trial of stimulation is performed to ensure good coverage of the patient's pain. Once final placement is determined, the leads are secured to the interspinous ligament, and the fascia is closed. Strain relief loops are made in the subcutaneous space and the leads are tightly secured to the fascia. This lead is then connected to a lead extender that is tunneled percutaneously to permit connection to an external pulse generator for the trial period.

Following a successful trial, the midline incision is re-opened and the percutaneous trial leads are cut and removed by a non-sterile assistant. The permanent leads are then tunneled to the chosen site for the implanted pulse generator. This may be in the subcutaneous fat of the flank or abdomen, depending on the preference of the patient and surgeon.

Awake versus Asleep Placement

Recent debate has emerged regarding whether electrodes are best placed with awake examination of the patient intraoperatively versus the use of general anesthesia and neuromonitoring. Awake placement allows for direct confirmation in the operating room that the paresthesias cover the region of the patient's pain. Surgeons who advocate for asleep placement argue that certain patients have physical and mental comorbidities that preclude awake surgery. Utilizing their fluoroscopy from a prior percutaneous trial to guide localization, electromyography and somatosensory evoked potentials are used to tailor placement. Testing is performed in a similar fashion to the awake patient, utilizing a standard screener box, but utilizing a significantly lower frequency, in the 5–10 Hz range. Each column of the lead is activated independently and the EMG response pattern is evaluated visually for symmetry. Some published reports show efficacy equal, and perhaps superior, to that of awake placement. One potential drawback of this method is the lack of direct patient feedback or the ability to detect unpleasant radicular stimulation when the patient is asleep. Unintended radicular stimulation is frequently the amplitude-limiting factor in SCS, and is typically detectable when the patient is awake during surgery, allowing for repositioning of the electrode. Patients under a general anesthetic would not be able to report such adverse stimulation.

Pivot Points

1. Spinal cord stimulation may be achieved with cylindrical leads placed percutaneously or with paddle-type leads implanted via a laminotomy.
2. The location of the patient's pain dictates the best level of the spinal cord to stimulate, typically T8-T12 for lower extremity pain.
3. Debate persists as to whether awake or asleep placement is best.

Aftercare

Following successful implantation of a paddle-type lead, patients are typically monitored for signs of development of any neurologic deficits for a brief period of time postoperatively. The external pulse generator is programmed to provide coverage of the region of pain and they are discharged home. During the trial period, some advocate placement on oral antibiotics. Patients are instructed on dressing changes for the lead exit site, as it is not uncommon to have serosanguinous drainage postoperatively.

Complications and Management

The common complications related to spinal cord stimulator placement are similar to those for other neurostimulators, related to the device itself. Infections affecting the pulse generator or the lead may require surgical removal of the device, as antibiotics often will not adequately treat the infection. Infection may be related to initial device placement, replacement of the implanted pulse generator, or it may be related to skin breakdown and erosions long after any surgery. Thus, it is important to implant these devices where there will be adequate tissue coverage and to encourage diligent monitoring on the part of the patient for any signs of skin changes following implantation. Pain in the device pocket may also cause significant distress to the patient and may require repositioning.

Lead damage may cause shorts or open circuits, leading to difficulty with programming. This occasionally will require lead or lead extender replacement.

While more common with percutaneous leads, it is still possible for paddle-type leads to migrate or lose ideal coverage. Lateral movement of the lead may cause uncomfortable chest wall stimulation. Often, adjustment of programming may aid in obtaining optimal coverage while minimizing side effects, but, on occasion, revision of the lead may be required.

> **Oral Boards Review—Complications Pearls**
>
> 1. Any sign of wound infection should be evaluated promptly and treated with antibiotics to prevent involvement of the SCS hardware.
> 2. If hardware infection is suspected, prompt removal of all involved hardware should be considered.

Evidence and Outcomes

There have been several case series and two recent larger clinical trials, including a randomized, controlled trial enrolling 60 patients, that have shown a significant reduction in pain from diabetic neuropathy and significant improvement in quality of life. These trials have had limitations, including a lack of control group or blinding and small sample size. The longest follow-up of these trials has showed durable reduction of pain by > 50% in 42% of patients at 1 year and 36% of patients at 5 years of follow-up. However, 80% of the patients enrolled in the study continued to use their stimulator, showing some continued benefit. Increasing objective severity of painful diabetic neuropathy at the time of implantation was associated with higher risk of treatment failure, particularly for patients with evidence of large sensory fiber involvement.

Further Reading

1. Kumar K, Toth C, Nath RK. Spinal cord stimulation for chronic pain in peripheral neuropathy. *Surgical Neurol.* 1996;46(4):363–369.
2. Bouhassira D, Wilhelm S, Schacht A, et al. Neuropathic pain phenotyping as a predictor of treatment response in painful diabetic neuropathy: Data from the randomized, double-blind, COMBO-DN study. *Pain.* 2014;155(10):2171–2179. doi:10.1016/j.pain.2014.08.020.
3. Tesfaye S, Vileikyte L, Rayman G, et al. Painful diabetic peripheral neuropathy: consensus recommendations on diagnosis, assessment and management. *Diabetes Metab Res Rev.* 2011;27(7):629–638. doi:10.1002/dmrr.1225.
4. Slangen R, Faber CG, Schaper NC, et al. A trial-based economic evaluation comparing spinal cord stimulation with best medical treatment in painful diabetic peripheral neuropathy. *Pain.* 2017;18(4):405–414. doi:10.1016/j.jpain.2016.11.014.
5. Pluijms WA, Slangen R, Van Kleef M, Joosten EA, Reulen JPH. Increased contact heat evoked potential stimulation latencies in responders to spinal cord stimulation for painful diabetic polyneuropathy. *Neuromod Technol Neural Interface.* 2014;18(2):126–132. doi:10.1111/ner.12188.
6. Pluijms WA, Slangen R, Bakkers M, et al. Pain relief and quality-of-life improvement after spinal cord stimulation in painful diabetic polyneuropathy: a pilot study. *Br J Anaesthesia.* 2012;109(4):623–629. doi:10.1093/bja/aes251.
7. van Beek M, Slangen R, Schaper NC, et al. Sustained treatment effect of spinal cord stimulation in painful diabetic peripheral neuropathy: 24-month follow-up of a prospective two-center randomized controlled trial. *Dia Care.* 2015;38(9):e132–e134. doi:10.2337/dc15-0740.

8. Duarte RV, Andronis L, Lenders MWPM, Vos CC. Quality of life increases in patients with painful diabetic neuropathy following treatment with spinal cord stimulation. *Qual Life Res.* 2015;25(7):1771–1777. doi:10.1007/s11136-015-1211-4.
9. van Beek M, Geurts JW, Slangen R, et al. Severity of neuropathy is associated with long-term spinal cord stimulation outcome in painful diabetic peripheral neuropathy: five-year follow-up of a prospective two-center clinical trial. *Dia Care.* 2017;41(1):32–38. doi:10.2337/dc17-0983.
10. de Vos CC, Rajan V, Steenbergen W, van der Aa HE, Buschman HPJ. Effect and safety of spinal cord stimulation for treatment of chronic pain caused by diabetic neuropathy. *J Dia Complic.* 2009;23(1):40–45. doi:10.1016/j.jdiacomp.2007.08.002.
11. Slangen R, Schaper NC, Faber CG, et al. Spinal cord stimulation and pain relief in painful diabetic peripheral neuropathy: a prospective two-center randomized controlled trial. *Dia Care.* 2014;37(11):3016–3024. doi:10.2337/dc14-0684.
12. Daousi C, Benbow SJ, MacFarlane IA. Electrical spinal cord stimulation in the long-term treatment of chronic painful diabetic neuropathy. *Dia Med.* 2005;22(4):393–398. doi:10.1111/j.1464-5491.2004.01410.x.
13. de Vos CC, Meier K, Zaalberg PB, et al. Spinal cord stimulation in patients with painful diabetic neuropathy: A multicentre randomized clinical trial. *Pain.* 2014;155(11):2426–2431. doi:10.1016/j.pain.2014.08.031.
14. van Beek M, van Kleef M, Linderoth B, van Kuijk SMJ, Honig WM, Joosten EA. Spinal cord stimulation in experimental chronic painful diabetic polyneuropathy: delayed effect of high-frequency stimulation. *Eur J Pain.* 2016;21(5):795–803. doi:10.1002/ejp.981.
15. Tesfaye S, Watt J, Benbow SJ, Pang KA, Miles J, MacFarlane IA. Electrical spinal-cord stimulation for painful diabetic peripheral neuropathy. *Lancet.* 1996;348(9043):1698–1701. doi:10.1016/S0140-6736(96)02467-1.

Cluster Headache

Emily Lehmann Levin

16

Case Presentation

The patient is a 25-year-old man who presents with headaches. The headaches may occur up to 8 times per day. They typically last 15 to 30 minutes. When they first started, they occurred only in summer months, but over the last 2 years, they have been without remission. Pain is isolated to the right half of the head and is associated with scleral injection and tearing of the right eye. These headaches have not responded to topiramate, lithium, or verapamil. He initially had relief with inhaled oxygen, although that has waned. He underwent a trial of occipital nerve stimulation one year ago but did not tolerate the paresthesias and was concerned about activity limitation to avoid migration of the leads.

Questions

1. What is the likely diagnosis?
2. What diagnoses are important to exclude?
3. What is the most appropriate imaging modality?
4. What is the appropriate treatment algorithm?

Assessment and Planning

This presentation is consistent with trigeminal autonomic cephalgia, specifically cluster headache, given the characteristics and demographic. The diagnosis is clinical, based on the International Classification of Headache Disorders II criteria; strictly unilateral episodic head pain, associated with ipsilateral scleral injection, tearing, rhinorrhea, and nasal congestion, facial sweating, ptosis, and miosis. It is more common in males. Patients with episodic cluster headaches will have short-lived periods of pain, occurring 1 to 10 times per day, with attacks separated by pain-free periods lasting at least 1 month. Those with chronic cluster headache may evolve from episodic and have symptoms lasting more than 1 year without remissions longer than 1 month.

It is important to exclude other pain syndromes, such as trigeminal neuralgia or migraine headaches. Trigeminal neuralgia does not have the autonomic features that trigeminal autonomic cephalgia classically does; in a patient who presents with tearing and scleral injection that accompanies the bouts of pain, cluster headache should be a prime consideration. Migraines and cluster headaches may be difficult to differentiate from one another. There are no laboratory values that are helpful in the diagnosis. An MRI or CT of the brain, particularly focusing on the hypothalamus and pituitary, may be useful to exclude a cause for secondary cluster headache, including vascular lesions, tumors, infectious or inflammatory etiologies. PET studies during an attack have shown posterior hypothalamic activation, although this has been used more for research than for diagnostic purposes.

While the exact pathophysiology of cluster headache is not known, it is believed to involve the trigeminal nerve and ganglion, with autonomic dysfunction and vascular irritability. Oxygen and parenteral triptans are first-line acute treatments. Corticosteroids have been shown to provide short-term relief from episodic attacks, although the attacks will typically recur as the medication is tapered. Long-term, evidence-based preventive agents include topiramate, verapamil, and lithium. Valproic acid has some supporting data as well, and it is thought to be useful in those who also suffer from migraines.

Surgery is limited to those patients that have persistent, chronic cluster headache with a minimum of three attacks per week, despite treatment with at least three preventative agents.

Questions

1. How does one choose a treatment for cluster headache?
2. When is surgical treatment appropriate?

Decision Making

For individuals with cluster headache, episodes may be so severe as to lead to suicidal ideation. Thus, it is important to recognize the disorder and initiate treatment with both preventative agents and acute therapies, typically starting with corticosteroids and verapamil. For an individual with chronic, daily headaches, one would run through each of the preventative agents in sequence. Once a patient has had an adequate trial of at least three agents, more interventional modalities may be considered.

Interventional treatments may be categorized as neuromodulatory or ablative. Occipital nerve blocks and stimulation have both been shown to be effective for the prevention of cluster headaches in small studies. Injection of corticosteroid around the greater occipital nerve has provided significant short-term benefit, as well. Although botulinum toxin injections have shown efficacy for chronic migraine, the data is lacking for cluster headaches.

Deep brain stimulation of the posterior hypothalamus arose from the autonomic symptoms and circadian rhythmicity noted in cluster headache, as well as anatomic and radiographic studies showing specific changes in the hypothalamus in patients with cluster headache. Guidelines have been published for patients in whom the benefits of hypothalamic DBS are thought to outweigh the risks. Typically, these include clear diagnosis of cluster headache, with the chronic form lasting at least 2 years. The patient must have inadequate relief with prophylactic and short-term abortive therapy. Many centers also include inadequate relief or inability to tolerate occipital nerve stimulation.

Surgical Procedure

Deep brain stimulation of the posterior hypothalamus has been shown to be effective in the treatment of chronic cluster headache. As in deep brain stimulation for movement disorders, accurate targeting relies on stereotactic coordinates, microelectrode recording, and intra-operative testing for therapeutic window. The most commonly reported target is that of the Franzini group: in AC-PC coordinates 2 mm lateral, 3 mm posterior, and 5 mm caudal to the MCP, ipsilateral to the side of pain. This target is located in the posterior hypothalamus, at the level of the subthalamic nucleus and red nucleus, and is based on early PET studies showing activation of this area during attacks.

Frame-based stereotaxy is usually used to provide for accurate placement. Low-dose sedation may be used. Antibiotics are administered. A pre-operative high-definition MRI is fused to an in-frame CT or MRI and a pre-coronal trajectory is planned. This trajectory should avoid significant vascular structures or passage through the ventricle. A rigid guide cannula is inserted from a standard paramedian burr-hole, aligned with the chosen trajectory. Microelectrode recording may be performed, although the electrographic signature of this region is not well characterized. Previous reports describe neurons with regular, infrequent firing, low amplitude, and low frequency (less than 20 Hz). The caudal border of the target region is identified by electrical silence (the interpeduncular cistern) or the characteristic firing of the red nucleus, depending on patient anatomy and trajectory. It is not advised to advance further should electrical silence be encountered due to the risk of vascular injury.

The microelectrode may then be withdrawn and the treatment electrode placed. Macro-stimulation is then performed to evaluate for side-effects. Typically, side effects, such as oculomotor deviations and a feeling of impending doom, are seen at greater than 4 V. Once there is satisfactory placement of the electrode, the guide cannula is removed and the electrode is secured to the skull.

Following successful placement of the brain electrode, it is connected to a subcutaneous internal pulse generator. Typical stimulation parameters for chronic stimulation are 180 Hz, 60-microsecond pulse width, with amplitude ranging from 0.7 to 3V in a voltage-controlled system.

Pivot Points

1. Programming of the deep brain stimulator to provide effective treatment of cluster headache requires patience and accurate recording of headache diaries by the patient.
2. Typical programming involves titration of monopolar stimulation up to just below the side-effect threshold and monitoring for headache improvement over the course of weeks.

Aftercare

Following successful implantation of the deep brain stimulation system, patients will typically receive imaging to confirm the placement of the electrode and to serve as a baseline should any lead migration occur. The patient is monitored overnight for neurologic changes and for pain and blood pressure management.

Complications and Management

Despite theoretical concerns regarding the fragility of the hypothalamus, there have been no reported complications specific to this target. The potential complications of deep brain stimulation are typical, no matter the target. Bleeding, infection, and device malfunction or malposition are the most worrisome complications. Asymptomatic hemorrhages surrounding the lead occur in approximately 5% of patients, with less than 1% of patients having a clinically significant hemorrhage. Infection occurs in approximately 5% of patients and must be treated early and aggressively. Limited superficial skin infections may be treated with antibiotics alone, but deeper infection requires removal of the involved hardware.

Oral Boards Review—Complications Pearls

1. Careful blood pressure management at the time of brain penetration is critical to the avoidance of intraparenchymal hemorrhage.
2. Any sign of wound infection should be evaluated promptly and treated with antibiotics to prevent involvement of the DBS hardware.
3. If hardware infection is suspected, prompt removal of all involved hardware is usually required.

Evidence and Outcomes

Cluster headache may typically be managed medically, and so it is quite uncommon to come to surgery. As such, the evidence for deep brain stimulation for the treatment of cluster headache is limited to a small number of individual case reports with more than a year follow-up, covering fewer than 50 patients. From 2003 until 2010, no formal blinded trials had been reported, although several patients had inadvertent device inactivation, resulting in a return of attacks. In 2010, Fontaine et al. published the only randomized, placebo-controlled, double blind trial with 11 patients. The blinded periods were only 1 month each and failed to show significant improvement in symptoms. However, during the 1-year un-blinded extension, there was a significant decrease in the number of attacks and significant improvement in patient satisfaction. When considering all published evidence, approximately 50 to 60% of reported patients implanted have a significant response to hypothalamic DBS.

Further Reading

1. Akram H, Miller S, Lagrata S, et al. Optimal deep brain stimulation site and target connectivity for chronic cluster headache. *Neurology*. 2017;89(20):2083–2091. doi:10.1212/WNL.0000000000004646.
2. Piacentino M, D'Andrea G, Perini F, Volpin L. Drug-resistant cluster headache: long-term evaluation of pain control by posterior hypothalamic deep-brain stimulation. *World Neurosurgery*. 2014;81(2):442.e11–442.e15. doi:10.1016/j.wneu.2013.01.130.
3. Franzini A, Messina G, Cordella R, Marras C, Broggi G. Deep brain stimulation of the posteromedial hypothalamus: indications, long-term results, and neurophysiological considerations. *Neurosurgical FOCUS*. 2010;29(2):E13. doi:10.3171/2010.5.FOCUS1094.

4. Sillay KA, Sani S, Starr PA. Deep brain stimulation for medically intractable cluster headache. *Neurobiol Dis*. 2010;38(3):361–368. doi:10.1016/j.nbd.2009.05.020.
5. Fontaine D, Lazorthes Y, Mertens P, et al. Safety and efficacy of deep brain stimulation in refractory cluster headache: a randomized placebo-controlled double-blind trial followed by a 1-year open extension. *J Headache Pain*. 2009;11(1):23–31. doi:10.1007/s10194-009-0169-4.
6. May A. Hypothalamic deep-brain stimulation: target and potential mechanism for the treatment of cluster headache. *Cephalalgia*. 2008;28(7):799–803. doi:10.1111/j.1468-2982.2008.01629.x.
7. Starr PA, Barbaro NM, Raskin NH, Ostrem JL. Chronic stimulation of the posterior hypothalamic region for cluster headache: technique and 1-year results in four patients. *J Neurosurg*. 2007;106(6):999–1005. doi:10.3171/jns.2007.106.6.999.
8. Franzini A, Ferroli P, Leone M, Broggi G. Stimulation of the posterior hypothalamus for treatment of chronic intractable cluster headaches: first reported series. *Neurosurgery*. 2003;52(5):1095–1101. doi:10.1227/01.NEU.0000057698.29634.D6.

Postherpetic Neuralgia of the Trigeminal Nerve (Trigeminal Tractotomy-Nucleotomy)

Zoe Teton and Ahmed M. Raslan

17

Case Presentation

A 79-year-old man sought care after a 7-year history of profound left-sided facial pain, particularly at the ophthalmic division of the trigeminal nerve, resulting from facial herpes zoster (shingles). He reported dull, aching background pain and episodic sharp, burning pain that was exacerbated by light touch. Previous treatments consisted of oral pregabalin and left supraorbital nerve stimulation, both of which had provided minimal pain relief. Neurological examination results were non-focal.

In the case of this patient, with a diagnosis of medically refractory postherpetic neuralgia (PHN), a decision was made to perform a left-sided computed tomography (CT)-guided trigeminal tractotomy-nucleotomy (TR-NC) with the patient awake. However, during the procedure, the patient was unable to tolerate the facial pain caused by the CT scanner headrest. After aggressive premedication and numerous attempts to reposition and pad the patient's face, the procedure was aborted. A decision was then made to proceed with an intraoperative CT-guided TR-NC with the patient under general anesthesia and use of somatosensory and motor-evoked potentials of the extremities and of the lower cranial nerves.

Questions

1. In what instances would you use trigeminal tractotomy as opposed to peripheral ablation?
2. Which diagnoses are the best candidates for trigeminal tractotomy?
3. What conditions are on the differential for PHN?

Assessment and Planning

The trigeminal or gasserian ganglion, located in Meckel's cave of the petrous temporal bone, contains pseudounipolar neurons. These neurons extend distal projections to the face, from nearly the vertex of the head to above the angle of the jaw and posteriorly to just into the auricle. There are three central nuclei that the central processes segregate to: (1) the mesencephalic nucleus, where proprioceptive fibers synapse; (2) the chief sensory nucleus in the pons, where light touch, pressure, and vibration are conveyed; and (3) the spinal nucleus, which carries pain and temperature fibers. From the spinal nucleus, the pain and temperature fibers decussate in the brainstem and travel in the ventral trigeminothalamic tract to ventral posteromedial nucleus (VPM) of the thalamus (13).

In the medulla, the descending trigeminal tract is dorsal to the spinal trigeminal nucleus at the level of the craniocervical junction. Sensory inputs from the head carried by cranial nerves V, VII, IX, and X also travel in the descending trigeminal tract and join the spinal nucleus. Within the descending trigeminal tract, there is topographical organization of the three trigeminal divisions. The spinal trigeminal nucleus extends from the pons down to C2 and has three subdivisions: (1) the nucleus oralis between the pons and medulla, (2) the nucleus interpolaris, (3) nucleus caudalis. The nucleus caudalis extends from the medullospinal junction down to C2 and has cytoarchitecture and neurochemistry similar to the substanstia gelatinosa of the spinal cord, highlighting it as a pain and temperature processing area. Lesioning of the entire nucleus caudalis at the dorsal root entry zone (DREZ) represents a more extensive version of the trigeminal nucleotomy, and it is performed via open approach after suboccipital craniectomy and C1 hemilaminectomy (12). Here, however, the focus is on the percutaneous procedure of TR-NC, which can be considered a "mini caudalis DREZ."

From a technical perspective, the location of the trigeminal tract shifts lateral from caudal to rostral, as such the trigeminal tract at C1 is more medial to its location at the craniocervical junction (Figure 17.1).

TR-NC is an effective operation in conditions where peripheral ablation would not be effective or could exacerbate the condition. Also, it is an effective procedure when pain is due to involvement of multiple cranial nerves such as cancer pain of the tongue or the face. Bilateral trigeminal V3 pain that is not a candidate for microvascular decompression (MVD) would be a good candidate for TR-NC given the risk of severe masticatory muscle weakness if peripheral ablation is contemplated (4, 5, 11, 13).

Patients falling into the following diagnoses can be considered good candidates for TR-NC: cancer- or tumor-related craniofacial pain, trigeminal neuropathic pain post-stroke pain, PHN, glossopharyngeal neuralgia, and geniculate neuralgia. However,

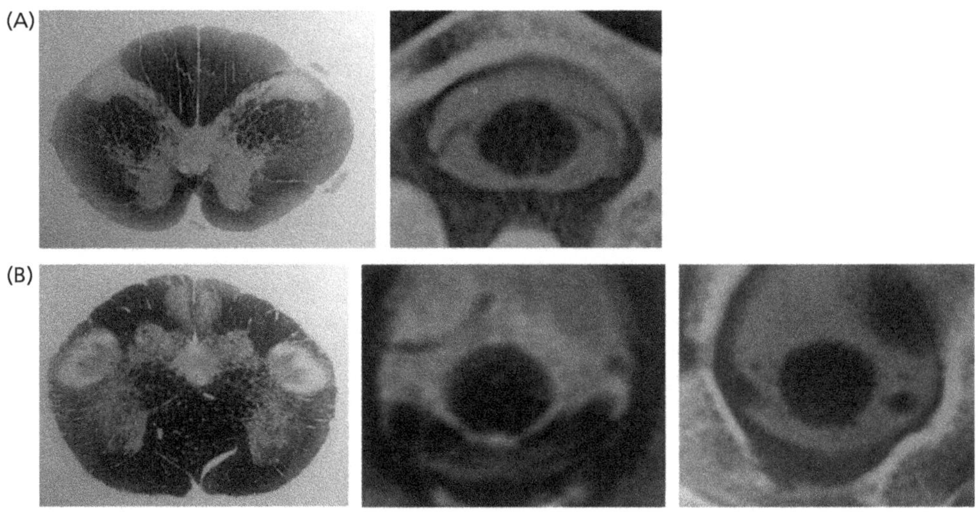

Figure 17.1. Pre-operative diagnostic work-up. A) Trigeminal tract at C1. B) Trigeminal tract at C0.

Anesthesia dolorosa may not be an ideal indication for TR-NC, as it requires an extensive lesioning of the trigeminal nucleus, which would not be possible with this needle-based approach (6).

Questions

1. Where is the spinal trigeminal nucleus located?
2. How does the trigeminal tract shift as you move from caudal (C1) to its location at the craniocervical junction?
3. Where does the nucleus caudalis extend to and from within the spinal trigeminal nucleus?

Oral Boards Review—Diagnostic Pearls

1. Trigeminal tractotomy is an effective operation in conditions where peripheral ablation would not be effective or could exacerbate the condition. The primary diagnoses that are good candidates for this procedure are trigeminal neuropathic pain, craniofacial cancer pain, glossopharyngeal or geniculate neuralgia, PHN, and post-stroke pain.
2. Lesioning of the entire nucleus caudalis at the DREZ represents a more extensive version of the trigeminal nucleotomy and is performed via open approach after suboccipital craniectomy and C1 hemilaminectomy. This chapter focuses on the less invasive, percutaneous TR-NC or "mini-caudalis DREZ."
3. The target of TR-NC is the lateral descending trigeminal tract and nucleus caudalis of the spinal trigeminal nucleus, located in the posterolateral aspect of the cervicomedullary junction. It is accessed between the occiput and C1.

Decision Making: Pros and Cons of Different Approaches and Intraoperative Considerations

CT-guided percutaneous ablation of the upper spinal cord for pain, including CT-guided TR-NC, now constitutes the most commonly used tractotomy-nucleotomy method. Percutaneous tractotomy is performed under local anesthesia, and needle position is verified by the awake patient after stimulation-induced paresthesia of the face. The introduction of intraoperative imaging, which is safe for patients under general anesthesia, enabled percutaneous CT-guided procedures to be performed in anesthetized patients (1). In the case described, performing the procedure under local anesthesia was not possible because of the extreme facial allodynia and hyperalgesia that the patient experienced in the prone position. Lateral positioning is an option, but direct prone positioning with the head in slight flexion is often preferred in order to ease anatomical guidance of the needle entry site and trajectory of the needle tip into the spinal cord. Conscious sedation or monitored anesthesia was not considered because the patient might move during the procedure, and any head movement while the tip of the electrode is in the upper spinal cord could result in complications such as hemiparesis or hemiplegia. In instances in which a full open caudalis DREZ procedure is not indicated (as in the present case), a percutaneous intraoperative CT-guided tractotomy-nucleotomy with intraoperative neuromonitoring can be performed for added safety. It can be argued that in patients for whom the anatomical target is very well characterized, such as the trigeminal tract, a lesion can be made without verification from the awake patient provided that real-time intraoperative verification of the electrode position is possible.

A CereTom CT scanner, which is specifically designed for cranial imaging and not spinal imaging, was used in this case. The physique of this patient (a long and thin neck) was such that use of the CereTom CT scanner in 3-point fixation was favorable. If patient physique is less favorable, a scan board designed to fit in the CereTom CT scanner may be necessary. If possible, the use of a whole-body or spine scanner such as the O-arm (Medtronic Inc., Minneapolis, MA) or BodyTom (Samsung Corp., Seoul, South Korea) is recommended for CT-guided tractotomy-nucleotomy procedures.

In select patient populations, careful lesion creation can be highly effective in providing immediate and long-lasting pain relief, with minimal adverse effects, lower cost, and shorter hospital stays. Although modulatory or pharmacologic treatments may be favored over ablative procedures, ablative procedures should be considered for patients with economic or logistic limitations that make intrathecal infusions challenging. Ablative TR-NC is effective in patients with craniofacial pain syndromes who wish to undergo a less invasive procedure than open craniotomy and caudalis DREZ.

Questions

1. What is the target of TR-NC and how is it accessed?
2. What intraoperative imaging scanners should be used in these cases?
3. What are the major complications associated with this procedure?

Surgical Procedure

The patient first undergoes lumbar puncture for injection of intrathecal contrast such as 300 iohexol (Omnipaque, GE Health Care). This is performed under local anesthetic while the patient is in the pre-operative holding area. Care must be taken to properly label the local anesthetic and contrast, so as to prevent inadvertent intrathecal local anesthetic injection. The patient then is kept in slight Trendelenberg position for 30 to 45 minutes. During that period, the patient is transported to the CT suite, and general anesthesia is induced. The patient is positioned prone on the CT table, with the head resting on a foam headrest, with care taken to keep the head neutral or in slight flexion. Often, monitoring somatosensory or motor-evoked potentials is not helpful due to the electrical artifact produced by the radiofrequency generator during lesioning. The procedure can be performed with a wide bore CT, be it in the diagnostic or operating suite, to avoid collision of the electrode with the scanner.

An initial localization CT is taken, centered on the craniocervical junction, from the foramen magnum to the caudal aspect of C1. Care is taken to avoid any metal fillings or dentures in the mouth that would create imaging artifact; typical slice thickness is 1–1.25 mm. The planned entry point into the skin, between the occiput and C1, is identified, and the distances from the skin to the dura and skin to the cord pia are

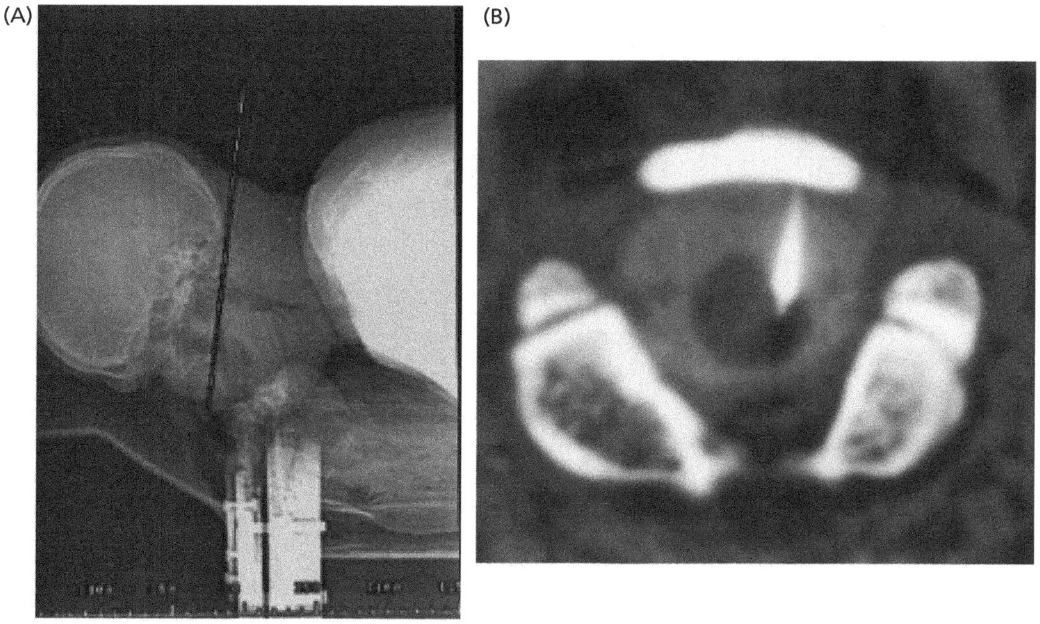

Figure 17.2. Surgical diagnostic evaluation and electrode placement. A) Lateral skull XR demonstrating placement of tractotomy electrode at craniocervical junction. B) Trigeminal tractotomy-nucleotomy lesion location.

measured. The target is identified, typically two-thirds of the distance from the midline to the equator of the spinal cord, which targets the trigeminal tract dorsally and the nucleus caudalis ventrally. The skin-to-dura distance is marked on the introducer cannula for the Levin-Cosman cordotomy electrode system (Cosman Medical, Burlington, MA). The electrode depth is adjusted to project 3 mm from the introducer metal cannula. The laser of the CT scanner is used to mark the entry point on the skin, and the site is prepped and draped sterilely. Serial CT scans are used guide the tip of the introducer needle to target. Once the subarachnoid space is entered, impedance, as measured by the Radionics RFG-3C generator (formerly Radionics Inc.), is 300–400 ohms. As the spinal cord is entered, impedance should increase to over 1000 ohms. After correct cannula positioning is confirmed on CT, the stylet is removed and the electrode introduced. Another scan is used to confirm positioning (Figures 17.2 and 17.3).

Sensory stimulation is performed at 50 Hz up to 0.1 V, which results in tachycardia, suggesting pain. Motor stimulation at 2Hz should show no motor activity in the ipsilateral leg. Generally, two tandem lesions are made. Given that TR-NC lesioning can be very painful, and that pain severity correlates directly with temperature used, lower lesion temperatures of 55 degrees are recommended for up to 120 seconds if the procedure is to be done awake. Higher lesion temperatures for shorter duration (similar to cordotomy parameters), such as up to 80 degrees for 60 seconds, also can be used.

Under general anesthesia, sensory stimulation is not possible, therefore anatomic verification using CT scan and electrophysiologic verification using motor stimulation are performed instead.

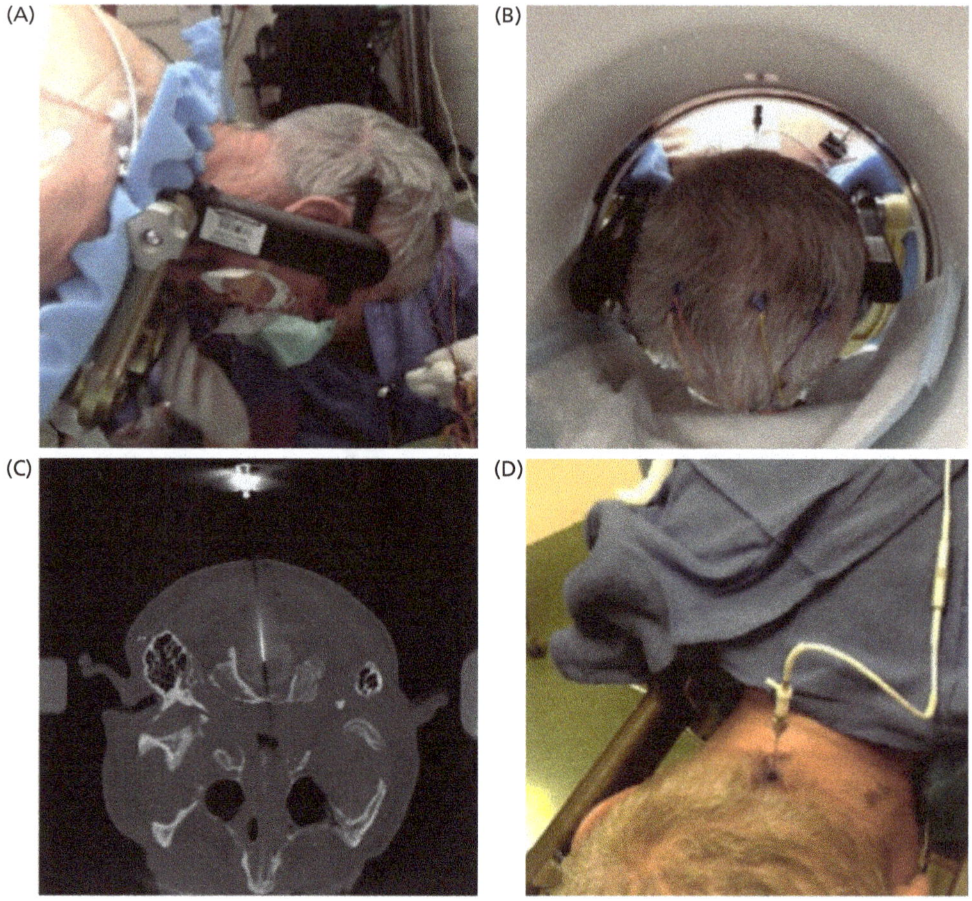

Figure 17.3. Steps of a percutaneous trigeminal tractotomy-nucleotomy performed using intraoperative CT and general anesthesia.

A) The patient is placed in rigid 3-point fixation in the prone position with the head flexed. The skull clamp is placed as inferiorly as possible to allow the plane of the CT scanner to reach C-2. B) The percutaneous needle is inserted 2 cm lateral to the midline between C-1 and the foramen magnum. Under CT guidance, it is directed to the trigeminal tract of the trigeminal nucleus, two-thirds of the distance from the midline to the equator of the spinal cord. C) The final position of the electrode tip is approximately 3 mm anterior to the dorsal surface of the cord and 6 mm lateral from the midline. D) Impedance is then assessed to ensure proper positioning of the electrode within the spinal cord and 2 lesions are made.

Source: Thompson EM, Burchiel KJ, Raslan AM. Percutaneous trigeminal tractotomy-nucleotomy with use of intraoperative computed tomography and general anesthesia: report of 2 cases. *Neurosurgical Focus.* 2013;35(3):E5. Reprinted with permission.

Oral Boards Review—Operative Management Pearls

1. The typical target identified in TR-NC is two-thirds of the distance from the midline to the equator of the spinal cord. This will target the trigeminal tract dorsally and the nucleus caudalis ventrally.
2. The pre-measured skin-to-dura distance should be marked on the introducer cannula for cordotomy electrode system. The electrode depth should be adjusted to project 3 mm from the introducer metal cannula, and serial CT scans should be used to guide the tip of the introducer needle to the target.
3. Impedance on entering the subarachnoid space will be 300–400 ohms. As the spinal cord is entered, this number will increase to over 1000 ohms.

Pivot Points

1. If the patient's pain level tolerates it, TR-NC can be performed awake, in the prone position, with CT guidance. The neurosurgeon just needs to ensure that the lower lesioning temperatures for a longer time period are used, as this period can be painful to the awake patient.
2. If the patient is experiencing severe facial pain, the more invasive nucleus caudalis DREZ procedure can be performed as well, as opposed to the CT-guided procedure under general anesthesia.

Aftercare

After lesioning, the needle with the electrode is removed and a final scan is obtained to examine the cord for any tract or contrast-penetration. Post-operatively, the patient should be observed in the intensive care unit for serial neurologic exams overnight. Typically patients discharge home the next day.

Complications and Management

The most commonly reported adverse effect is transient ataxia of the ipsilateral upper extremity from edema of the dorsal spinocerebellar tract. Reported rates range from 5 to 10%. Ipsilateral or contralateral paresthesia due to involvement of the dorsal column or the spinothalamic tract are also possible side effects of the TR-NC procedure. Motor weakness is very unlikely, due to the ventral location of motor pathways at the level of the craniocervical junction.

Oral Boards Review: Complications Pearls

1. Ataxia of the ipsilateral upper extremity is the most common adverse effect. This is due to edema of the dorsal spinocerebellar tract and is very often transient.

2. Paresthesias, contralateral or ipsilateral to the side of the lesion, may also occur due to involvement of the dorsal column or spinothalamic tract during the tractotomy procedure.
3. Motor weakness is very unlikely, due to the ventral location of motor pathways at the site of the lesioning (craniocervical junction).

Evidence and Outcomes

The majority of outcome literature comes from the experiences of Drs. Kanpolat and Raslan (5, 1112). Kanpolat's largest series describes 65 patients over a follow-up period of 20 years: 21 with atypical facial pain; 13 with craniofacial malignancies; 17 with vagoglossopharyngeal neuralgia; and the remainder with geniculate neuralgia, PHN, cluster headache, anesthesia dolorosa, or failed trigeminal neuralgia. Kanpolat et al. report that early pain relief was obtained in 84% of patients, with a statistically significant immediate postoperative reduction in Visual Analog Scale score of 5.4. (12) The best results were obtained in the vagoglossopharyngeal neuralgia patients and geniculate neuralgia patients. Nineteen of 21 patients with atypical facial pain achieved pain relief and 11 of 13 patients with craniofacial or oral cancer pain achieved relief. In these 65 patients, the procedure was performed 73 times. There were no mortalities, but there was a 6% rate of transient ataxia due to large lesions affecting the spinocerebellar tract. All instances of ataxia these resolved within 2 weeks.

Raslan et al. reported on 10 patients who underwent TR-NC in 2008 (5) for the treatment of facial pain secondary to malignancy. They are reported along with a cohort of 41 patients who underwent unilateral cordotomy (lesioning of the spinothalamic tract between C1 and C2) for localized body pain. These 10 patients underwent the procedure while awake, and underwent sensory test stimulation at 100 Hz for 0.1 ms until severe ipsilateral face or throat pain was reproduced at less than 0.5 V. This aided in confirmation of proper electrode placement. Voltage threshold above 0.5 V or sensory response in a limb implies inaccurate electrode placement. Motor test stimulation at 2 Hz for 0.1 ms also was performed. If no motor response was obtained in the ipsilateral hemibody other than local contraction of the neck musculature with voltages above 1 V, then lesioning was performed. Two lesions were performed: the first typically at 45 degrees for 180 seconds, and then the second at 55 degrees for 120 seconds. This article provides useful parameters for relevant CT measurements (i.e., mean skin-to-dura distance is 51.4 mm) and impedance (mean 1272.9 ohms). Mean age was 52.1 yr, with time from pain onset to surgical procedure ranging from 1 to 9 months. Ninety-eight percent of patients reported no pain or partial satisfactory pain relief post-procedure, with the rate still high at 80% at 6 months. Average sleeping hours and mean Karnofsky Performance Score both increased. Since this large initial case series, the Raslan team have transitioned to performing the procedure under general anesthesia.

In a large review of ablative procedures for cancer pain, seven papers were identified that examined the use of TR-NC in the treatment of facial pain from cancer. In the single open label prospective study included, the authors found a sustained pain relief of 80% at 6 months. The other six studies were case series, and the number of patients treated with TR-NC was still relatively low at just 50 overall. There was no level I or II evidence for the therapy (5).

Further Reading

1. Sjogvist O: Studies on pain conduction in the trigeminal nerve. A contribution to the surgical treatment of facial pain, in Acta Psychiatr Neural Scand Suppl XVII. *Helsingfors: Mercators Tryckeri*. 1938; pp 93–122.
2. Spiller W, Martin E: The treatment of persistent pain of organic origin in the lower part of the body by division of the anterolateral column of the spinal cord. *JAMA*. 1912;**58**:1489–1490.
3. Hitchcock E: Stereotactic trigeminal tractotomy. *Farmatsiia*. 1970;**19**:131–135.
4. Raslan AM: Percutaneous computed tomography-guided radiofrequency ablation of upper spinal cord pain pathways for cancer-related pain. *Neurosurgery*. 2008;**62**:226–233; discussion 233–224.
5. Raslan AM, Cetas JS, McCartney S, Burchiel KJ: Destructive procedures for control of cancer pain: the case for cordotomy. *J Neurosurg*. 2011;**114**:155–170.
6. Thompson EM, Burchiel KJ, Raslan AM: Percutaneous trigeminal tractotomy-nucelotomy with use of intraoperative computed tomography and general anesthesia: report of 2 cases: *Neurosurg Focus*. 2013;**35**(3):E5.
7. Falconer MA: First and second division trigeminal neuralgia treated by intramedullary trigeminal tractotomy. *Proc R Soc Med*. 1954;**47**(4):299–300.
8. Crue BL, Carregal EJA, Felsoory A: Percutaneous stereotactic radiofrequency trigeminal tractotomy with neurophysiological recording. *Stereotact Funct Neurosurg*. 1972;**34**:389–397.
9. Fox JL: Intractable facial pain relieved by percutaneous trigeminal tractotomy. *JAMA*. 1971;**218**:1940–1941.
10. Hitchcock E: Stereotactic trigeminal tractotomy. *Ann Clin Res*. 1970;**2**:131–135.
11. Kanpolat Y, Deda H, Akyar S, Caglar S, Bilgic S: CT-guided trigeminal tractotomy. *Acta Neurochirurgica*. 1989;**100**(3–4):112–114.
12. Kanpolat Y, Kahilogullari G, Ugur HC, Elhan AH: Computed tomography-guided percutaneous trigeminal tractotomy-nucleotomy. *Neurosurgery*. 2008;**63**(1 Suppl 1):ONS147–153; discussion ONS153–145.

Cingulotomy for Intractable Pain

Patrick J. Hunt, Patrick J. Karas, Ashwin Viswanathan, and Sameer A. Sheth

18

Case Presentation

A 64-year-old man with stage IV metastatic prostate cancer complains of excruciating back pain, which he describes as maximum on a visual analog scale. He has numerous known metastases to his thoracic and lumbar spine. He has undergone several trials of chemotherapy and is currently on a palliative regimen. He has also undergone palliative radiation to the bony metastases in his spine. He complains of back pain that is present both at rest and during activity, severely limiting his sleep and mobility. He denies the presence of pain radiating through his chest wall or down his legs. His MRI shows no pathologic fractures or neural compression, but he does have some narrowing of his spinal canal due to osteoblastic metastases. His wife and son, who accompany him to the appointment, mention that his mood is down, he has trouble sleeping, and despite being an avid sports fan, he shows no interest in the recent success of his favorite football team. His palliative care physician referred him to a neurosurgeon after he failed multiple regimens of oral analgesics and topical medications.

Questions

1. What are the standard pharmacologic treatments for chronic pain?
2. What are the options for surgical intervention in chronic pain?
3. How is the severity of chronic pain scored?
4. What clinical criteria must a patient meet prior to consideration for surgery for chronic pain?

Assessment and Planning

Roughly 10% of Americans suffer from chronic pain, with more than half of these patients describing their pain as maximum on pain measurement scales. The etiologies of chronic pain are numerous and diverse, making it difficult to treat this symptom consistently in all patients. First-line treatment of chronic pain includes numerous different classes of pharmacological drugs, commonly divided into nonopioid (e.g., nonsteroidal anti-inflammatory drugs) and opioid analgesics. However, many patients experience chronic pain refractory to first-line treatments. In addition, analgesics are often accompanied by adverse side effects and can induce tolerance, which may not be acceptable in many populations. In these patients, invasive, nonpharmacologic treatment options should be considered, including ablative surgeries such as anterior cingulotomy.

The goal of anterior cingulotomy is to create bilateral lesions at the junction of the anterior cingulate cortical gray matter and the subjacent cingulum white matter tract. Anterior cingulotomy for pain grew out of John Fulton's anterior cingulectomy procedures, used in the late 1940s as an alternative psychiatric surgery to decrease the morbidity and mortality seen in other psychiatric procedures of the time, such as frontal lobotomy. The advent of stereotactic techniques in the late 1940s and early 1950s permitted accurate, reproducible, less invasive alternatives to open resections. Ballantine applied these stereotactic techniques to perform cingulate ablations in the 1960s at the Massachusetts General Hospital, thus introducing the cingulotomy procedure. Over the next several decades, the cingulotomy yielded beneficial outcomes in psychiatric patients while avoiding significant adverse effects. Many of these early patients developed a decreased dependency on pain medications. In 1968, Foltz and White reported the first series of patients for which anterior cingulotomy was used to treat refractory chronic pain. Since that time, numerous case series have demonstrated the effectiveness of anterior cingulotomy in alleviating severe, pharmacologically intractable chronic pain.

The use of anterior cingulotomy has decreased in recent decades, largely due to advances in neuromodulatory alternatives such as intrathecal pumps, spinal cord stimulators, and deep brain stimulation. Chronic pain refractory to pharmacologic treatment merits consideration of surgical options such as intrathecal pumps and electrical neuromodulation. Cingulotomy is generally considered after failure of these nonlesioning, reversible interventions. In some situations, however, cingulotomy may be preferable to these options, including in patients too cachectic to tolerate an implant, those with advanced malignancies and short life expectancy, or for those who find that managing a device is too burdensome. Cingulotomy also offers the benefit of reducing the psychological or affective component of chronic pain.

Severe, intractable, chronic pain can arise secondary to many causes. The etiology of this pain is commonly categorized as cancer-related (tumor infiltration, treatment-related neuropathic pain, etc.) or non-cancer-related (post-traumatic neuropathic pain, atypical facial pain, diabetic neuropathy, phantom pain, etc.). Variation in etiology results in variable presentations in patients being evaluated for anterior cingulotomy. However, patients with chronic pain refractory to previous treatment and/or with a significant psychologic component to the pain may be candidates for this procedure.

Quantifying the patient's pain is important both in assessing the patient and evaluating surgical success. Several commonly used pain scales include the Visual Analog Scale (VAS), the 10-point Likert scale, and the McGill pain scale.

Neurosurgeons caring for patients with chronic pain must work closely with pain management specialists. Given the role of anterior cingulotomy in treating refractory chronic pain in late-stage cancer patients, close collaboration with oncologists and palliative care specialists is also often essential.

Oral Boards Review—Diagnostic Pearls

1. Surgeons performing pain procedures should work closely with pain specialists, oncologists, and/or palliative care teams for both pre-operative evaluation and post-operative long-term management.
2. Anterior cingulotomy may function by reducing the emotional reaction (i.e., affective dimension) to pain and therefore may be a good choice in patients with comorbid depression or anxiety.
3. Modern neuromodulatory interventions for pain, including intrathecal pumps, spinal cord stimulators, and deep brain stimulation, involve implantation of hardware that may not be cost effective in patients with end stage malignancies and refractory chronic pain. In addition, patients with chronic pain and comorbid chronic infection may not be good candidates for implantation of stimulation devices. These populations may benefit from anterior cingulotomy as a first-line invasive treatment.

Questions

1. What is the current theory for the pathophysiology of chronic pain?
2. Describe the neural pathways that play a role in the pathophysiology of chronic pain.
3. What are the differences between nociceptive and neuropathic pain?

Decision Making

The affective dimension of pain refers to the unpleasantness associated with pain. The anterior cingulate cortex is thought to play an important role in this facet of the pain experience. Experimental and functional imaging studies have demonstrated a direct role for the cingulate cortex in processing chronic pain. Interestingly, in vitro studies have demonstrated that excitatory synapses of the anterior cingulate cortex undergo long-term potentiation in response to injury. Moreover, this potentiation can continue in the absence of input from the peripheral nervous system, thereby implicating the anterior cingulate cortex in the generation of chronic pain. Thus, rather than changing the patient's ability to sense pain, modulating activity within the anterior cingulate cortex alters the patient's suffering, thereby providing relief.

Pain can be categorized as nociceptive or neuropathic pain. Nociceptive pain is caused by tissue damage and manifests as somatic (from the skin, muscles, etc.) or visceral (from the internal organs) pain. This damage is detected by peripheral nociceptors and passed on to pain processing brain centers by afferent sensory pathways. Nociceptive pain can often be well localized, although somatic pain is generally more easily localized than visceral pain. Causes of nociceptive pain include trauma-induced tissue damage, tissue compression, or destruction secondary to space-occupying neoplastic lesions, infection, or chemical irritation. The nature of nociceptive pain is dependent on the cause of the pain. This pain is often responsive to pharmacologic treatment but can prove to be intractable.

Neuropathic pain arises from an insult to a part of the nervous system itself. Causal lesions may be found anywhere from nerve fibers to cortical and subcortical pain processing centers (e.g., anterior cingulate cortex, thalamus) and often result in pain that is lancinating, burning, shooting, or tingling. Neuropathic pain is often associated with allodynia (perception of pain to a stimulus that does not usually cause pain) and hyperalgesia (perception of increased level of pain to a painful stimulus). Pathologies associated with neuropathic pain include post-stroke pain, thalamic pain, phantom limb pain, pain after spinal cord injury, and pain resulting from chronic neurological diseases like multiple sclerosis. This type of pain is often unamenable to chronic pharmacologic treatment, thus proving intractable.

Whether nociceptive or neuropathic, intractable pain can be treated with both neuromodulatory and lesioning procedures.

Questions

1. What are the commonly observed adverse events following anterior cingulotomy?
2. What permanent adverse events may be seen following anterior cingulotomy?
3. What is the effectiveness of anterior cingulotomy for chronic pain?

Surgical Procedure

Surgical ablation of the anterior cingulate cortex can be achieved with several methods, including radiofrequency ablation (RFA) or laser interstitial thermal therapy (LITT). RFA has been used for decades, whereas LITT is a relative newcomer, used for cingulotomy only within the past decade. No single method has been proven to be superior to the others, so surgeons should use the method with which they are most comfortable and familiar. Nonsurgical ablative procedures such as stereotactic radiosurgery (SRS) and focused ultrasound may also be used but have not been adequately studied for the application of anterior cingulotomy for chronic pain.

Prior to surgery, the anterior cingulate cortex should be localized using a preoperative stereotactic quality magnetic resonance image (MRI) scan. The anterior cingulate cortex lies within the medial aspect of the cerebral hemispheres and partially circumscribes the corpus callosum. Stereotactic planning can be performed using standard techniques. The choice of the stereotactic system (traditional frame, custom-printed frame, burr hole-mounted frame, robotic, frameless, etc.) is the surgeon's preference.

Targeting has varied across studies over the decades and is usually done based on anatomy rather than on a standardized coordinate system. The Y-coordinate (anterior-posterior; Figure 18.1) is the most variable across studies, ranging from 17.5 to 37.5 mm posterior to the anterior tip of the frontal horn of the lateral ventricle. In a meta-analytic review of lesion locations, Sharim and Pouratian showed that outcomes improved with more anterior lesion placement, within the range used in previous studies. Lesions closer to 17.5 millimeters posterior to the tip of the frontal horn tended to show better outcomes than those located more posteriorly. Interestingly, Steele and colleagues in Scotland found similarly improved outcomes with more anteriorly placed lesions in a series of patients with intractable depression treated by cingulotomy. The X coordinate

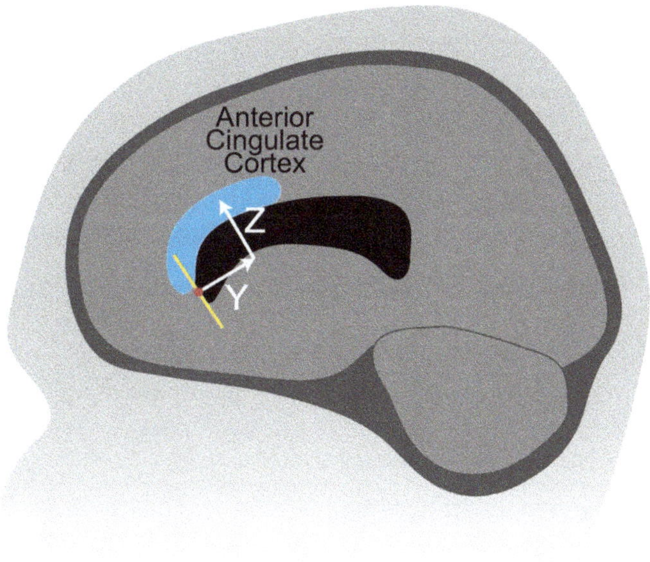

Figure 18.1. Targeting the Anterior Cingulate Cortex. Diagram of a mid-sagittal view of the brain. Targeting for cingulotomy procedures is usually accomplished based on anatomy rather than a standardized coordinate system such as the AC-PC (anterior commissure, posterior commissure) plane. Axes are determined by a line (yellow line) tangential to the furthest anterior tip of the frontal horn of the lateral ventricle (red circle). The Y axis projects perpendicular to this line (parallel to the roof of the lateral ventricle). The Z axis runs perpendicular to the Y axis, and is followed superiorly towards the cingulate gyrus. The X axis runs in and out of the page.

(medial-lateral) is typically 7–10 mm from the midline, within the mid-portion of the cingulate cortex. The Z coordinate (superior-inferior) is 5–10 mm above the roof of the lateral ventricle, near the border between the corpus callosum and cingulate cortex.

After skin incision, bilateral burr holes are created based on the stereotactic plan, and the dura is opened. Care should be taken to minimize cerebral spinal fluid loss during the procedure, as copious cerebral spinal fluid drainage can lead to brain shift and loss of stereotactic precision. Trajectories should be carefully chosen to avoid crossing blood vessels. Viswanathan et al. report their technique for lesioning the anterior cingulate gyrus using RFA with a radiofrequency probe with a 10 mm exposed tip. Once the probe is at target, it is heated to 80°C for 90 seconds. After cooling, the electrode is withdrawn 10 mm and a second lesion more dorsal is created.

MRI-guided LITT has also been used to create the cingulotomy lesion, as reported by Patel et al. In this procedure, the laser cannula/fiber assembly is placed to target using standard percutaneous stereotactic techniques and secured using a skull-mounted anchor bolt. The patient is then taken to the MRI scanner, where MRI thermography sequences are used to measure the temperature at every voxel within the chosen field of view. As the laser is turned on, the tissue heating can be visualized in real time, and the software calculates an estimate of irreversibly coagulated tissue based on temperature and duration.

RFA procedures can be performed under general anesthesia or local anesthesia/sedation, whereas LITT procedures are usually performed under general anesthesia to avoid movement in the MRI scanner.

Oral Boards Review—Management Pearls

1. Both RFA and LITT have been successfully used for cingulotomy. The choice is a matter of surgeon/patient preference.
2. Stereotactic technique is also a matter of preference, as this procedure can be performed with any of the acceptable stereotactic platforms.
3. The Y (anterior-posterior) coordinate of the target varies most significantly across previous studies, from 17.5 to 37.5 mm posterior to the tip of the frontal horn. There is some suggestion that more anterior location within this range may produce better outcomes.

Pivot Points

1. A patient who presents with intractable chronic pain, especially if there is a significant psychologic aspect to their pain, or if the patient suffers from a terminal illness, should be evaluated for anterior cingulotomy.
2. Close follow-up should evaluate for pain amelioration, adverse effects, and should involve collaboration with pain specialists.

Aftercare

Patients are observed in an inpatient setting following surgery and are generally discharged on post-operative day 1 in uncomplicated cases. A post-operative MRI or CT scan is recommended prior to discharge for evaluation of lesion site and volume and to detect potential complications. Serial neurologic exams should also be continued until discharge to detect early complications.

Complications and Management

Most commonly observed side effects resolve within days of the operation. Acute and usually temporary effects include headache, nausea, confusion, and vomiting. Because of the target location near micturition and lower extremity motor control regions, urinary incontinence and gait disorders have also been observed but also tend to resolve. Serious or permanent adverse events occur only in rare cases (<5% for each adverse event) and include seizures, intraparenchymal hemorrhage, personality changes (e.g., flat affect), and impairments in executive functioning, attention, visual-processing, or simple motor skills. Psychiatric symptoms such as paranoid ideations have also been reported in occasional cases. In many patients, impairments of executive function that are found within 3 months following ablation resolve by 12 months. However, other changes in cognition, such as impairments in spontaneous word production, focused attention, and design fluency have been found to remain impaired in some patients even 12 months after surgery.

Oral Boards Review—Complication Pearls

1. Common side effects are mild (e.g., headache, nausea, confusion, vomiting) and typically transient.
2. Serious adverse events can be permanent but are rare. These include behavioral changes, seizures, intraparenchymal hemorrhage, and motor deficits.
3. Because of the ablative nature of this procedure, hardware-related complications seen in neuromodulatory procedures, including lead fracture, infection, and erosion, are not relevant.

Evidence and Outcomes

A meta-analysis of 41 patients by Agarwal and colleagues found that pain improved by 50–100% on pain assessment scales. These outcomes were similar in both cancer-related and non-cancer cases.

The largest analysis (Sharim and Pouratian, mentioned previously) of patients undergoing anterior cingulotomy for the treatment of intractable chronic pain reviewed 224 surgical cases across 11 studies, including cases involving cancer-related as well as non-cancer-related pain. Of these patients, 67% (n = 149) reported significant pain relief in the immediate post-operative period. Notably, there was not a significant difference between those with cancer-related and non-cancer-related pain. Patients with cancer-related pain had shorter follow-up records on average, primarily due to disease-related death. However, in both cohorts combined, 65% (n = 53 of 82) of patients reported sustained pain relief 12 months after surgery (cancer: 67% [n = 6 of 9], non-cancer: 64% [n = 47 of 73]). Additionally, this report found that of the 10 reoperations, 8 provided significant pain relief or improved pain relief compared to the initial ablation. Of the 6 reoperation cases with 4 + weeks of follow-up, 4 (67%) patients sustained significant pain relief.

Anterior cingulotomy has demonstrated efficacy in ameliorating treatment-resistant chronic pain for over 60 years. The rise of effective neuromodulatory procedures, which are non-destructive and programmable/reversible, has led to an increase in these procedures over the past decade. However, in cases where pain is refractory to those therapies, ablation remains a valid option. Moreover, device-based therapies may not be appropriate for certain populations of patients with chronic pain, such as those with a short life expectancy due to advanced metastatic cancer, or those with chronic infection. In addition, cingulotomy may be preferable for patients with a significant psychological component to their pain.

Further Reading

Agarwal N, Choi PA, Shin SS, Hansberry DR, Mammis A. Anterior cingulotomy for intractable pain. *Interdisciplinary Neurosurg: Adv Techniques Case Management.* 2016; 6: 80–83.

Ballantine HT, Cassidy WL, Flanagan NB, Marino R. Stereotaxic anterior cingulotomy for neuropsychiatric illness and intractable pain. *J Neurosurg.* 1967; 26(5): 488–495.

McGovern RA, Sheth SA. Role of the dorsal anterior cingulate cortex in obsessive-compulsive disorder: converging evidence from cognitive neuroscience and psychiatric neurosurgery. *J Neurosurg*. 2016; 126(1): 132–147.

Nicolaidis S. Neurosurgical treatments of intractable pain. *Metabolism*. 2010; 59 Suppl 1: S27–S31.

Patel NV, Agarwal N, Mammis A, Danish SF. Frameless stereotactic magnetic resonance imaging-guided laser interstitial thermal therapy to perform bilateral anterior cingulotomy for intractable pain: feasibility, technical aspects, and initial experience in 3 patients. *Neurosurgery*. 2015; 11 Suppl 2: 17–25; discussion 25.

Sharim J, Pouratian N. Anterior cingulotomy for the treatment of chronic intractable pain: A systematic review. *Pain Physician*. 2016; 19(8): 537–550.

Sheth, SA, Neal J, Tangherlini F, Mian MK, Gentil A, Cosgrove GR, et al. Limbic system surgery for treatment-refractory obsessive-compulsive disorder: a prospective long-term follow-up of 64 patients. *J Neurosurg*. 2013; 118(3): 491–497.

Steele JD, Christmas D, Eljamel MS, Matthews K. Anterior cingulotomy for major depression: clinical outcome and relationship to lesion characteristics. *Biol Psychiatry*. 2008; 63(7): 670–677.

Viswanathan A, Harsh V, Pereira EA, Aziz TZ. Cingulotomy for medically refractory cancer pain. *Neurosurg Focus*. 2013; 35(3): E1.

Wang GC, Harnod T, Chiu TL, Chen KP. Effect of an anterior cingulotomy on pain, cognition, and sensory pathways. *World Neurosurg*. 2017; 102: 593–597.

Trigeminal Neuropathic Pain

Motor Cortex Stimulation

Nicholas C. Field and Julie G. Pilitsis

19

Case Presentation

A 65-year-old female presented to her primary care physician complaining of a severe persistent burning pain on the right side of her jaw following a tooth extraction. The procedure was 18 months ago and was complicated by an infection. Her dentist had assured her the pain would resolve once the infection was treated. The pain was stabbing and shocking in nature and was provoked with eating, speaking, or cold air. Initially, her primary care physician started her on an NSAID and eventually added gabapentin and narcotics. She continued to experience significant jaw pain and was referred to a neurologist who began treatment with carbamazepine. Despite initial relief with carbamazepine, the pain continued and she was diagnosed with trigeminal neuralgia. Magnetic resonance imaging (MRI) brain did not show vascular compression of the trigeminal nerve. She was subsequently referred to a neurosurgeon and underwent a percutaneous radiofrequency rhizotomy of the V3 branch of the trigeminal nerve.

She had initial pain relief; however, 6 months later, she experienced recurrent pain. Although the pain was in the same distribution, it was now constant and burning, rather than episodic. Detailed history and neurological examination by the neurosurgeon confirms a constant unilateral pain and burning sensation in the V3 distribution of the trigeminal nerve. There are no other focal findings on examination. The surgeon carefully reviews the patient's medical and surgical treatments to date.

Questions

1. What is the differential diagnosis?
2. What is the most appropriate imaging modality?
3. Has her neurologist exhausted all conventional treatments?
4. What other investigations should the neurosurgeon order prior to scheduling surgery?

Assessment and Planning

The differential diagnosis for craniofacial pain syndromes includes trigeminal neuralgia, trigeminal neuropathic pain, postherpetic neuralgia, anesthesia dolorosa, central neuropathic pain, and persistent idiopathic facial pain. The most common of these syndromes, trigeminal neuralgia, has an annual incidence of 4–13/100,000 per year and is more commonly reported in women. The majority of these cases are caused by microvascular compression of the trigeminal nerve at its entry into the pons. An MRI with a thin slice T2 gradient echo sequence can be used to assess for microvascular compression of the trigeminal nerve from its origin at the pons to the trigeminal ganglion at Meckel's cave.

However, due to the constant nature of her pain, the burning nature of the pain, and the presentation after rhizotomy, the functional neurosurgeon suspects the patient is suffering from trigeminal neuropathic pain.

Oral Boards Review—Diagnostic and Preoperative Pearls

1. Detailed history and physical examination is critical to differentiate between different craniofacial pain syndromes whose treatment may significantly differ.
   a. *Pain characteristics*. Pain can be distributed in distinct V1, V2, and V3 tracts similarly to TN, or located more diffusely.
   b. *Nerve injury*. Injury to the trigeminal nerve during sinus or dental surgery is a common precipitating event, as is facial trauma. Previous TN surgery may also predispose to neuropathic pain. Neuropathic pain may also occur due to chemotherapy, metabolic causes, and herpes virus.
2. Validated standardized tests, such as the Visual Analog Scale and the McGill Pain Questionnaire, are important diagnostic tools to assess the success of treatments and should be administered prior to any intervention, whether surgical or medical.
3. Preoperative psychological evaluation and discussion surrounding goals of care and realistic expectations are mandatory prior to undergoing any procedure.
4. MRI to rule out vascular compression of the trigeminal nerve should be performed. Brain MRI may also diagnose multiple sclerosis or thalamic strokes as other causes of trigeminal neuropathic pain.

Questions

1. How do these clinical and radiological findings influence surgical planning?
2. What intraoperative strategies can the surgeon use to decrease the risk of complications and improve outcomes?
3. What pre- and postoperative assessments should be used to judge the success of surgery?

Decision Making

The mainstay treatment of most cases of trigeminal neuralgia is medical management with carbamazepine, which may provide relief in upward of three-quarters of patients. However, the pain in some individuals may prove refractory. Multiple surgical procedures have been developed to treat these conditions, and range from microvascular decompression, a mainstay of trigeminal neuralgia treatment, to glycerol rhizotomies. Trigeminal neuropathic pain may also respond to carbamazepine or other neuropathic pain agents. Botulinum toxin may also be effective. Neuromodulation with peripheral nerve stimulation (PNS) or motor cortex stimulation (MCS) has also demonstrated impressive results. PNS has been particularly successful in treating pain in the distribution of V1 and V2 by stimulating the supraorbital and infraorbital nerves, respectively, as well as with occipital neuralgia. There are reports of treating V3 pain with ganglion stimulation, and we have anecdotal experience with peripheral V3 stimulation. First reported in 1991 by Tsubokawa et al., MCS is an effective treatment strategy for a range of chronic facial pain syndromes, particularly in the treatment of trigeminal neuropathic pain.

Prior to undergoing any procedure, validated pain scales such as the Visual Analog Scale and McGill Pain Questionnaire should be administered to establish a baseline pain score. A pain psychology assessment must be performed by an independent practitioner to evaluate the patient for depression, drug abuse, or other disorders that would prevent them from undergoing surgical treatment.

Questions

1. What diagnostic and intraoperative studies should be employed in order to achieve the safest and most successful outcome for the patient?
2. What conditions and patients are most suitable candidates for motor cortex stimulation?

Surgical Procedure

An fMRI should be performed in addition to an MRI for neuronavigation. Specifically, blood oxygen level–dependent imaging sequences acquired while the patient undergoes motor tasks, such as the hat task, will assist in the localization of the pre-central gyrus (Figure 19.1). MCS is a major procedure carried out under general anesthesia without motor blockade as a two-stage procedure. Stage one consists of the insertion of the electrode paddle, while stage two involves generator placement. In stage one, patients are positioned supine on a standard table with their head tilted to the contralateral side with the aid of a shoulder roll. A Mayfield pin system is used to stabilize the patient's head. Neuronavigation is carefully registered and its accuracy confirmed by using anatomical landmarks; it is subsequently used to identify the central sulcus. Antibiotics should be given within an hour prior to incision. A 5-cm linear incision is marked over the central sulcus, centered over the facial eminence. The patient is prepped and draped in the usual sterile fashion and a timeout is held. Local anesthetic is administered, after which the skin incision is made. The corresponding craniotomy should be large enough to accommodate the paddle electrode.

Somatosensory evoked potential (SSEP) recording of the median nerve is performed over the dura using the paddle electrode to detect the N20-P20 phase reversal, which aids in identifying the central sulcus (Figure 19.2). Once identified, the electrode is placed in the orientation of the precentral gyrus, centered over the facial eminence. Intraoperative cortical monitoring using the electrode can aid in localizing the facial eminence. The electrode is secured to the outer layer of the dura mater using silk suture (Figure 19.3). In order to identify the motor threshold, sedation may be lightened and motor cortex stimulation performed until facial muscle twitches are observed. This value is useful to avoid side effects during post-operative programming. Sedation should be deepened and the bone flap replaced and secured with titanium plates. The leads exit via

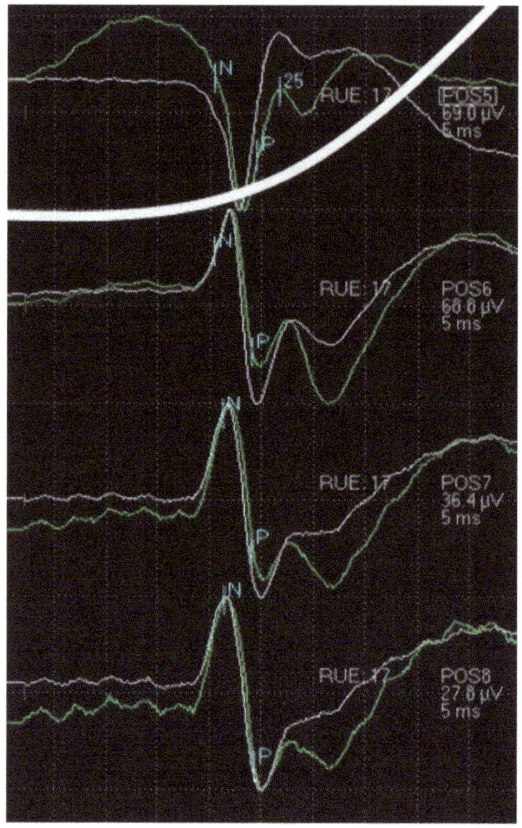

Figure 19.1. SSEP N20/P20 phase reversal recording used to identify the central sulcus (represented by the white line). Image courtesy of Impulse Monitoring.

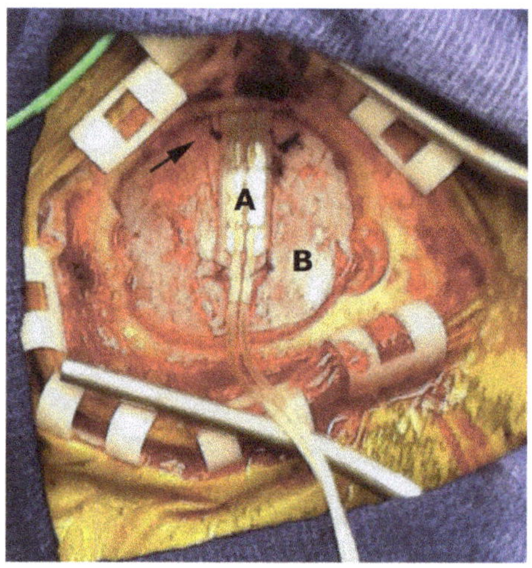

Figure 19.2. Intraoperative photograph of electrode placement (A) secured with silk ties (arrow) to the dura in the epidural space (B) during motor cortex stimulation procedure.

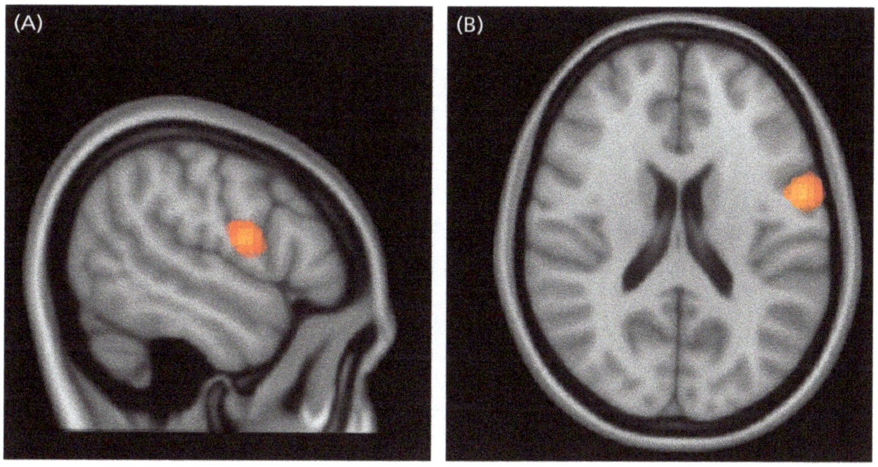

Figure 19.3. Functional magnetic resonance imaging can be used to understand the somatotopic arrangement of the motor cortex. The data can be integrated with intraoperative neuronavigation for stimulator targeting.

one of the burr-hole sites and are tunneled posteriorly out of a separate skin incision. Prior to closure of the craniotomy incision, extreme care should be taken to achieve hemostasis, and copious irrigation is necessary. The incision is then closed in deep and superficial layers.

Stage two of procedure typically occurs 7 to 10 days later following a successful trial. The patient should be positioned supine with a shoulder roll and the head rotated to the contralateral side. The generator is implanted inferior to the clavicle at the depth recommended by the specific manufacturer and the incision should be marked ahead of time. Prepping and draping should create continuous sterile field from the original incision along the neck and the ipsilateral superior chest so that all aspects of the stimulator system can be accessed, if necessary. Lead extensions connecting to the stimulator paddle are tunneled through the subcutaneous tissue from the cranial to the generator incision.

Oral Boards Review—Management Pearls

1. Preoperative and intraoperative localization of the somatotopic face region of the precentral gyrus using neuronavigation and SSEPs is critical.
2. An invasive procedure, motor cortex stimulation should be considered and only undertaken after medical management has failed.

Pivot Points

1. Investigations are ongoing to determine which patients will be the best responders to motor cortex stimulation. Potential factors that have been identified include opiate insensitivity and response to transcranial magnetic stimulation.

2. Few surgeons advocate for subdural placement of the electrode paddle; however, there are no randomized controlled trials comparing epidural versus subdural placement. Subdural placement may have a higher incidence of postoperative hemorrhage and a greater risk of postoperative seizure.
3. Some surgeons opt to implant the electrode and generator in one operation, thus decreasing the time spent under general anesthesia.
4. Pain reduction of greater than 50% is necessary to achieve during the stimulator trial before permanent implantation can be considered.

Aftercare

The post-operative course is similar to that of anyone undergoing a craniotomy, with the exception that the initial procedure is considered a trial prior to permanent implantation. Patients typically undergo a post-operative CT scan and receive peri-operative antibiotics for 1 day. Due to the elevated risk of seizure, we recommend 7 days of antiepileptic drug therapy. Patients should continue their current pain medication regimen in addition to post-operative medications, unless the team has a set algorithm to test response to the device. The chronic pain population often includes patients on high-dose narcotics, which should not be discontinued. Consultation with an acute pain service may be necessary if the patient requires continuous intravenous medications such as ketamine.

Programming of the stimulator is typically done on post-operative day 1. Parameters include amplitude (0.5–10 Volts), pulse width (45–450 μs), and frequency (25–130 Hz). In order to proceed with permanent implantation, pain reduction of greater than 50% without inducing side effects such as seizures or paresthesias must be achieved. Due to the risks of seizure, programming must occur in a setting where immediate seizure treatment and management can occur. Multiple case series have shown that temporary pain relief persists after the stimulation is stopped, so many surgeons use a cycling mode that alternates between periods of on- and off-stimulation. The same validated pain scales used preoperatively should be used to reassess the patient at the end of the trial. Patients typically require multiple programming sessions to achieve maximal results.

Complications and Management

The most commonly reported complication in the literature is seizure, which can occur intraoperatively or more commonly during the postoperative period during direct epidural cortical stimulation. Caution must be used during stimulator programming. Intraoperatively, these are typically treated with phenytoin.

Local wound infection is an unfortunate complication, which all measures should be taken to prevent as it typically requires the removal of all implanted hardware. Other complications include formation of an epidural hematoma.

Unusual complications have been reported after motor cortex stimulation and have included development of a painful supernumerary phantom limb, bilateral analgesia from unilateral stimulation, and development of new pain when stimulation is active.

Oral Boards Review—Complications Pearls

1. Intra-operative seizure may be induced by direct epidural motor cortex stimulation.
2. Epidural hematomas can occur following surgery, and patients should be monitored closely in the immediate preoperative period.
3. Hardware implantation carries an increased infection risk, and perioperative antibiotics and strict sterile technique are of utmost importance.
4. Post-operative seizure, particularly during the initial programming phase, is common. Programming should be performed in a clinic equipped for seizure management.
5. Decreasing efficacy of stimulation over time may require reprogramming of the stimulator.

Evidence and Outcomes

First reported as a treatment for trigeminal neuropathic pain in 1991, subsequent case series have continued to report the benefits of MCS. However, evidence supporting MCS from prospective clinical trials is still lacking.

With the advancement of imaging modalities, primarily MRI and intraoperative neuronavigational systems, the procedure has been continually refined. However, no agreed upon technique is uniformly practiced, including whether the electrodes are placed perpendicularly or parallel to the central sulcus, which leads to implant, and what the most appropriate stimulator settings are. Overall, MCS has shown promising results and few long-term complications in a wide variety of patients suffering from intractable trigeminal neuropathic pain. Enthusiasm has been tempered by relative inexperience with programming, which may lead to suboptimal results.

Further Reading

Brown JA, Pilitsis JG. Motor cortex stimulation for central and neuropathic facial pain: a prospective study of 10 patients and observations of enhanced sensory and motor function during stimulation. Neurosurgery. 2005 Feb 1;56(2):290–297. https://www.ncbi.nlm.nih.gov/pubmed/15670377

Henderson JM, Lad SP. Motor cortex stimulation and neuropathic facial pain. Neurosurg Focus. 2006 Dec;21(6):1–4. https://www.ncbi.nlm.nih.gov/pubmed/17341050

Monsalve, GA. Motor cortex stimulation for facial chronic neuropathic pain: a review of the literature. Surg Neurol Int. 2012; 3(Suppl 4): S290–S311. https://www.ncbi.nlm.nih.gov/pubmed/23230534

Nguyen JP, Lefaucher JP, Le Guerinel C, Eizenbaum JF, Nakano N, Carpentier A, Brugieres P, Pollin B, Rostaing S, Keravel Y. Motor cortex stimulation in the treatment of central and neuropathic pain. Arch Med Res. 2000 Jun 30;31(3):263–265. https://www.ncbi.nlm.nih.gov/pubmed/11036176

Rasche D, Ruppolt M, Stippich C, Unterberg A, Tronnier VM. Motor cortex stimulation for long-term relief of chronic neuropathic pain: a 10 year experience. Pain. 2006 Mar 31;12(1):43–52. https://www.ncbi.nlm.nih.gov/pubmed/16480828

Occipital Nerve Stimulation for Chronic Refractory Migraine

Cletus Cheyuo, Roy S. Hwang, and Julie G. Pilitsis

20

Case Presentation

A 34-year-old male presented to clinic with a 20-year history of headaches, which he described as originating in the occipital area and radiating anteriorly, with 10/10 intensity, with associated blurring of vision, nausea, vomiting, and sometimes slurred speech. He denied any known triggering and relieving factors. He has headaches 4 times per week and each episode of headache may last a couple days. Sometimes neck pain is associated. He had no relief of his headaches with narcotics, muscle relaxants, or non-steroidal anti-inflammatory drugs. He was evaluated by a neurologist who performed multiple bilateral greater occipital nerve blocks with bupivacaine and steroids, which provided transient relief of the headaches. Since the patient had transient relief of his headaches with bilateral greater occipital nerve blocks, he was referred to a neurosurgeon for neurosurgical treatment options.

Questions

1. What is the diagnosis?
2. What additional studies are required?
3. Does he have chronic or episodic headaches, and is his condition intractable?

Assessment and Planning

The patient was diagnosed with chronic migraine without aura. The neurosurgeon considered the patient a potential candidate for occipital nerve stimulation (ONS) due to the refractory nature of his migraines. The patient underwent neuropsychological evaluation.

Oral Boards Review—Diagnostic Pearls

1. Migraines are recurrent headache attacks lasting 4–72 hours, with characteristics of unilateral location, pulsating quality, and moderate or severe intensity. They can be aggravated by routine physical activity and associated with nausea, photophobia, and phonophobia.
2. A patient has chronic migraines if headache symptoms are present more than 15 days per month, of which 8 of those days constitute the definition

of migraine. Episodic headaches are less than 15 days per month. These symptoms must occur for greater than a 3 month duration.

3. Intractability is not currently definitively defined, but failure of three of the following preventative medications are considered diagnostic for intractability: beta-blockers, anticonvulsants, tricyclic antidepressants, flunarizine or candesartan, and Botox.

Decision Making

Neuropsychological evaluation showed no contraindication. The patient underwent trial implantation with 100% improvement in his headache pain and wished to proceed with permanent implant of stimulator device. X-ray images from the trial were used for placement of the permanent device.

Oral Boards Review—Management Pearls

1. A clinical diagnosis of intractable chronic migraines should be determined prior to consideration of ONS.
2. Patients should undergo a thorough neuropsychological evaluation prior to implantation to rule out comorbid psychiatric disorders as well as tolerability for the procedure and aftercare.
3. A trial of ONS should be performed.

Surgical Procedure

The patient was brought to the operative suite and induced under general endotracheal anesthesia. He was prone and his face placed into a prone view head holder. Hair was clipped from the inion to the retroauricular region bilaterally. He was prepped and draped in sterile fashion with the entire planned path of the occipital lead in the sterile field, to prevent the needle from penetrating the skin under the drapes. The patients armed were kept at his sides and battery placement planned on right flank.

The incision sites were infiltrated with local anesthetic with epinephrine. One 3 cm incision was made at the midline. The subcutaneous tissue was undermined at the level of the fascia to allow for placement of strain relief loop. A battery site was prepared with dissection 1 cm below the skin to allow for a rechargeable battery. A passing incision was made approximately at the level of the scapula to allow for an additional strain relief loop. A shunt passer was introduced to connect all three incisions. Tuohy needles were then used to advance percutaneous 8-contact leads at the level of the fascia. The dens was used as the landmark of where on the skull the leads should be placed. Once placement mimicked the trial, each of the electrodes was then secured using 2-0 silk stitches tied around the electrode arrays in three point fixation to the fascia. A strain relief loop was made. The lead was tunneled to the skip incision where an additional strain relief loop was made and then ultimately the lead was tunneled to the internal programmable generator (IPG). Once connected, IPG connections were found to be adequate through

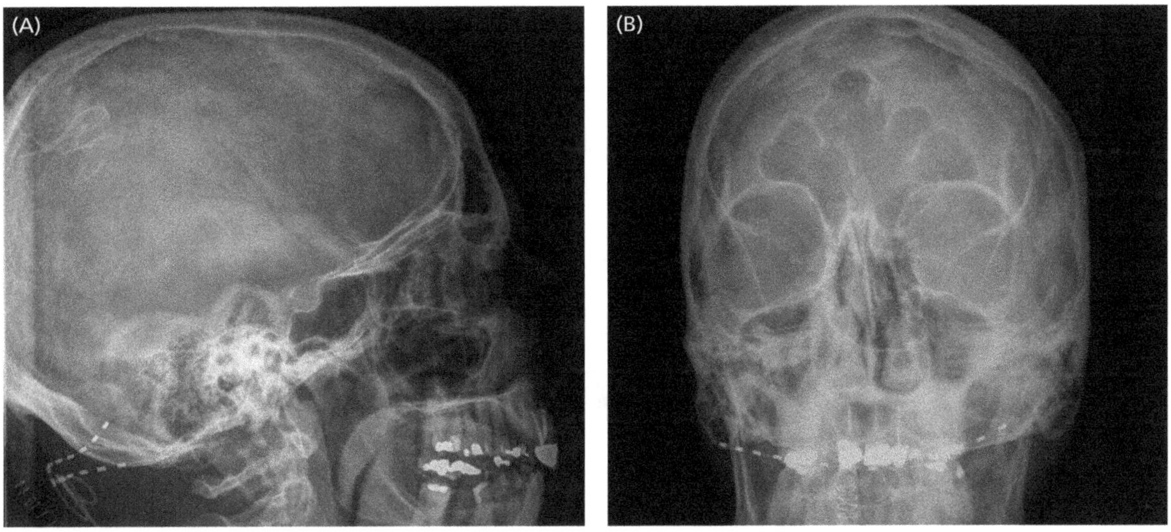

Figure 20.1. X-ray of skull, lateral view (left) and AP view (right), demonstrating bilateral occipital nerve stimulators.

an impedance check and was anchored to the tissue below. After copious irrigation, the incisions were closed in an interrupted fashion.

Aftercare and Follow Up

At the end of the surgical procedure, the patient was extubated and sent to the recovery room. Postoperative skull radiographs optimal placement (Figure 20.1). He was discharged home with 2 week follow up. At follow up, the patient reported significant reduction in headaches with improved quality of life. The surgical incision was healing well and the sutures were removed. At 6 weeks follow up the patient continued to have excellent improvement in his headache symptoms.

Complications and Management

At 7 months postoperatively, the patient presented to the outpatient clinic with complaints of erosion of stimulator electrodes through the skin as well as an electrical sensation radiating from the back of his head. The left occipital nerve stimulator electrode tip was superficial and likely the cause of the electrical sensation the patient was experiencing. Cultures were negative and there was no evidence of infection. He underwent left occipital nerve stimulator lead revision and continued to have excellent control of his headaches.

Oral Boards Review—Complications Pearls

1. It often takes 3–6 months for maximum clinical improvement for patients with ONS; therefore patients should be conservatively managed if there is a lack of clinical improvement in symptoms and hardware appears in optimal position.

2. The most common adverse effects of ONS is hardware issues, migration, erosion, and infection.
3. Meticulous technique is critical in avoiding hardware failure. Anchoring the leads and creating strain relief loops helps prevent migration. Placement should avoid pressure points such as behind the superior part of the external ear to avoid skin breakdown from eyeglass irritation. Post-operatively, patient should avoid extreme movements until the leads have undergone fibrosis.

Evidence and Outcomes

A recent systemic review and meta-analysis of ONS for chronic migraine by Chen et al.[1] found five randomized controlled clinical trials (RCTs)—PRISM study,[2] ONSTIM study,[3] Silberstein et al. 2012,[4] Sara and Marchioretto 2012,[5] and Slotty et al. 2014.[6] These RCTs included three industry-sponsored, multicenter, parallel group trials (PRISM study, ONSTIM study, and Silberstein et al. 2012) and two single-center crossover trials (Serra and Marchioretto 2012 and Slotty et al. 2014). The PRISM study (published only as a conference abstract) was a multicenter, parallel-group study that included 63 patients for ONS versus 62 patients for sham. Using "days with prolonged (≥ 4 hours) moderate or severe headache" as an outcome measure, the PRISM study reported a prespecified subgroup analysis that showed a trend in favor of patients without medication overuse (ONS vs. sham, reduction of 5.9 vs. 2.6 migraine days/month) compared with patients with medication overuse (ONS vs. sham, reduction of 5.0 vs. 4.8 migraine days/month).[2] The ONSTIM study was a multicenter, parallel-group with three arms: ONS (n = 28) versus sham (n = 16) versus medication management (n = 17). The ONSTIM study showed that ONS provided significant mean reduction in headache days at 3 months (ONS 6.7 ± 10.0; sham 1.5 ± 4.6; and medication management 1.0 ± 4.2). ONS also resulted in significant mean reduction in overall pain intensity (0–10 scale) at 3 months (ONS 1.5 ± 1.6; sham 0.5 ± 1.3; and medication management 0.6 ± 1.0). In addition, ONS resulted in a significant mean change in Migraine Disability Assessment grade at 3 months (ONS 0.4 ± 0.8; sham, not reported; and medication management: 0.0 ± 0.0).[3] Silberstein et al. conducted a multicenter, parallel group—ONS (n = 105) versus sham (n = 52). Patient-reported percentage headache pain relief at 3 months was significantly higher in the ONS group (ONS 42% versus sham 17%). In this study, mean reduction in Migraine Disability Assessment scores at 3 months were also better in the ONS group compared to sham.[4] Sara and Marchioretto conducted a single-center, crossover, ONS "on" vs. "off" study (n = 29). ONS "on" was associated with significant reductions in median headache days per week at 1 month and median headache severity (0–10 scale) at 1 month.[5] Slotty et al. conducted a single center, crossover study, comparing suprathreshold versus subthreshold versus no stimulation (n = 8). This study reported a significant improvement in pain was observed in favor of suprathreshold stimulation compared to subthreshold stimulation (1.98 ± 1.56 vs. 5.65 ± 2.11). Pain was also significantly improved under subthreshold stimulation compared to no stimulation (5.65 ± 2.11 vs. 8.45 ± 0.99).[6]

In addition to these RCTs, multiple institutions have shown that ONS provides very good to excellent pain control. These studies have also reported excellent patient satisfaction. Zhou et al. followed 24 patients for 4.9 years after implantation of peripheral nerve stimulators for control of medically refractory headaches. They demonstrated significant reduction in total pain index and self-rated treatment satisfaction was excellent in 54% of the patients, very good or good in 42%, and fair in 4%. None of the patients developed any complications.[7] Similarly, Miller et al. investigated the long-term efficacy, functional outcome, and safety of ONS in an uncontrolled, open-label, prospective study of 53 with intractable chronic migraine. This study demonstrated response rate of 34.3% to 66.7% depending on the type of headache. The mean subjective patient estimate of improvement was 31.7% and the adverse event rate was reported as favorable.[8] Lead migration remains one of the most common complications after peripheral nerve stimulator implantation. In a retrospective analysis of 18 patients who underwent ONS for refractory headaches, Pittelkow et al. described utilization of a 2-point anchoring technique with a tension-relief loop and use of ultrasound for lead placement as ways to decrease lead migration.[9]

Further Reading

1. Chen YF, Bramley G, Unwin G, Hanu-Cernat D, Dretzke J, Moore D, Bayliss S, Cummins C, Lilford R. Occipital nerve stimulation for chronic migraine: a systematic review and meta-analysis. PLoS One. 2015 Mar 20;10(3):e0116786.
2. Lipton RB, Goadsby PJ, Cady RK, Aurora SK, Grosberg BM, et al. PRISM study: occipital nerve stimulation for treatment-refractory migraine [abstract PO47]. Cephalalgia. 2009;29: 30. doi: 10.1109/IEMBS.2009.5335024.
3. Saper JR, Dodick DW, Silberstein SD, McCarville S, Sun M, Goadsby PJ; ONSTIM Investigators. Occipital nerve stimulation for the treatment of intractable chronic migraine headache: ONSTIM feasibility study. Cephalalgia. 2011 Feb;31(3):271–285.
4. Dodick DW, Silberstein SD, Reed KL, Deer TR, Slavin KV, Huh B, Sharan AD, Narouze S, Mogilner AY, Trentman TL, Ordia J, Vaisman J, Goldstein J, Mekhail N. Safety and efficacy of peripheral nerve stimulation of the occipital nerves for the management of chronic migraine: long-term results from a randomized, multicenter, double-blinded, controlled study. Cephalalgia. 2015 Apr;35(4):344–358.
5. Serra G, Marchioretto F. Occipital nerve stimulation for chronic migraine: a randomized trial. Pain Physician. 2012 May-Jun;15(3):245–253.
6. Slotty PJ, Bara G, Kowatz L, Gendolla A, Wille C, Schu S, Vesper J. Occipital nerve stimulation for chronic migraine: a randomized trial on subthreshold stimulation. Cephalalgia. 2015 Jan;35(1):73–78.
7. Zhou L, Ashkenazi A, Smith JW, Jen N, Deer TR, Zhou C. Long-term clinical outcome of peripheral nerve stimulation for chronic headache and complication prevention. *Anesth Pain Med.* 2016;6(4):e35983.
8. Miller S, Watkins L, Matharu M. Long-term outcomes of occipital nerve stimulation for chronic migraine: a cohort of 53 patients. *J Headache Pain.* 2016;17(1):68.
9. Pittelkow TP, Pagani-Estevez GL, Landry B, Pingree MJ, Eldrige JS. Occipital neuromodulation: A surgical technique with reduced complications. *Pain Physician.* 2016;19(7):E1005–E1012.

Complex Regional Pain Syndrome Diagnosis and Surgical Management

Roy S. Hwang, Claire Collison, and Julie G. Pilitsis

21

Case Presentation

A 61-ear-old female farmworker suffered a left shoulder injury from heavy lifting four years prior and required a subsequent rotator cuff repair. She developed persistent burning pain on the left upper extremity with neck and shoulder pain that radiated intermittently on the inner arm towards the elbow. This pain was much worse than her prior preoperative pain symptoms. On examination, she had significant allodynia of the entire left upper extremity and noted weakness and decreased range of motion of the proximal and distal left upper extremity. Her left upper extremity appeared symmetric to her right upper extremity; however, there was noted loss of hair on the left. MRI imaging of the shoulder and cervical spine were obtained. The shoulder showed chronic injuries while the cervical spine showed no significant stenosis of the neuroforamen or central canal. She has undergone extensive physical and occupational therapy without much progress due to increasing pain and decreasing range of motion.

Questions

1. What is the likely diagnosis? And what subtype?
2. What event in her history is typically seen in patients with this diagnosis?

Assessment and Planning

She was diagnosed with complex regional pain syndrome (CRPS) type I, formerly reflex sympathetic dystrophy. She underwent several steroid injections on the shoulder with some success with a sympathetic block. However, based on her physical and occupational therapy assessments, it was determined that she required further intervention in order for further functional improvement. The next step was a cervical spinal cord stimulator trial, which provided greater than 50% improvement in her symptoms.

Oral Boards Review—Diagnostic Pearls

1. Since CRPS is a clinical diagnosis, the history and clinical presentation are the most critical and should be focused on. Often patients have pain symptoms out of proportion to their inciting event and not in a particular nerve distribution.

2. There are two types, I and II, which are based on the absence or presence of nerve injury, respectively. CRPS I typically occurs from an inciting event such as a fracture, an elective orthopedic surgical procedure, or a minor trauma to an involved extremity. Incidence of occurrence ranges from 3 to 30% in reported literature.[1]
3. CRPS can be diagnosed according to the Budapest consensus guidelines for clinical diagnosis.[2]
   a. Continuing pain, which is disproportionate to any inciting event.
   b. At least one symptom in three of the four categories: sensory, vasomotor, sudomotor/edema, motor/trophic
   c. At least one sign at the time of evaluation in two or more categories: sensory, vasomotor, sudomotor/edema, motor/trophic
   d. No other diagnosis to exclude
4. It is important to rule out other potential causes of extremity pain, and a complete work-up of the central and peripheral nervous system pathology or musculoskeletal pathologies is recommended.

Questions

1. What is the overall goal of therapy?
2. What guidelines are available for diagnosis of CRPS?
3. What additional work-up should be performed?
4. What interventional options are available?

Decision Making

The patient had initiated functional restoration management with physical therapy and medication management with anti-depressant and anti-convulsant therapy. She also underwent several sympathetic nerve blocks with some relief but decreasing effectiveness over time. The patient underwent trial of cervical SCS with > 50% improvement reported in pain symptoms. The patient was then counseled on permanent implantation of a cervical spinal cord stimulator.

Questions

1. What are the indications for surgical management? What conservative treatments should be exhausted prior to consideration of SCS?
2. What pre-operative imaging should be obtained prior to implantation? What pre-operative history and work-up should be performed prior to surgical implantation?

Surgical Procedure

Percutaneous Electrode Placement

We perform our percutaneous placement under general anesthesia. We position prone in a prone view head holder on a Wilson frame and perform neuromonitoring with EMG.

The cervico-thoracic area and battery site locations are prepped. Using intraoperative fluoroscopy we locate the T3-4 interspace for cervical placement and the L2-3 interspace for thoracic placement and make a small stab incision just inferior to our entry point. Much of the literature discusses using a T12-L1 entry point. We prefer to go below the conus if possible. For cervical placement, we insert our introducer needle under fluoroscopic guidance in a near vertical plane using either a hanging drop or loss of resistance technique to confirm we were in the epidural space. We guide the percutaneous lead under direct fluoroscopic until we are in accordance to the stimulator trial placement. We do modify this position based on where the sweet spot was during the trial to have that spot in the middle of the lead, whenever possible. In CRPS cases when one side is affected, we place a single lead. We check EMG to ensure placements, looking for deltoid or trapezius activation on the side of placement. We make another incision in the flank on the side the patient prefers to create a subcutaneous pocket for the battery. Once the lead(s) are in final position, we remove the stylet and the introducer needle, and we suture the anchor down to the underlying fascia, using silk suture; a shunt passer is used to tunnel from the battery pocket. Extensions are used in cases where there is not enough lead length to comfortably make strain relief loops at the anchor and battery site. The battery is sutured in place and impedance are checked. The incisions are irrigated, and the wounds are then closed.

Epidural Paddle Placement

Cervical paddle placement is rare in CRPS and is generally reserved for cases when there is a significant component of axial neck pain that is not adequately treated with the trial. We perform our cervical SCS surgery under general anesthesia with intraoperative neuromonitoring. After induction and intubation, the patient is positioned prone over a Wilson frame in a Mayfield head holder with the neck in neutral position. The suboccipital area is shaved, prepped, and a 5-cm cervical incision centered over C1 is made. The occipital bone and the inter-laminar spaces between C1 and C3 are exposed. Then we use an instrument such as a Woodson and Penfield #4 to dissect the epidural space from occipital to the top of C3. Spinous process and some lamina are often removed. Then a surgical paddle is placed in a retrograde fashion centered over the C2 body and the odontoid, in the midline. Intraoperative EMG is used to confirm that the laterality of the electrode contacts stimulate the left and right sides, respectively, by EMG activation in the upper extremities. A cranial plate is used as an anchor to the occiput with a piece of gel foam in between the plate and the lead. We make an incision on the lower back on the side of the patient's preference just above the belt line for our generator placement in a subcutaneous pocket. A tunneler is used to pass the wires of the electrode caudally, which is tunneled through an intermediary incision in the thoracic area and then connected to an extension lead. A release loop is left at the thoracic area and then the lead extensions are connected to the impulse generator. We anchor the generator using silk suture to the subcutaneous tissue and the fascia. The cervical incision is closed in layers with 0 Vicryls and 2-0 Vicryls.

For our thoracic SCS placement we similarly position prone under general anesthesia on a Wilson frame with a standard prone view head rest. Our paddle is placed centered on the pre-operative SCS trial sweet spot. We mark a midline incision to perform a laminotomy one or two interspaces below the target area, depending on the lead we plan to place, and mark a low-back incision accordingly to the patient's preference generally above the belt line. We generally perform a minimal laminotomy of the lamina above the interspace we target using the drill, Kerrison rongeurs, and curettes. We remove the ligamentum flavum to expose the thecal sac below and pass our epidural paddle within this space. We use intraoperative fluoroscopy to confirm positioning. Intraoperative EMG is used to confirm that the laterality of the electrode contacts stimulate the left and right sides, respectively, by EMG activation of the abdominal muscles and lower extremities. All other portions are done similarly to our cervical SCS placement except that in this location, we do not need extension leads to connect the generator to the electrode paddle.

Oral Boards Review—Management Pearls

1. Overall management should aim for functional restoration through desensitization, reactivation, flexibility and strength training, ergonomics, and functional rehabilitation.[2]
2. Medication management includes calcium channel blockers, NMDA receptor agonists, alpha-adrenergic antagonists, opioids, and anti-depressants. Class I or II level evidence or efficacy of the above is lacking.[3] One clinical study for the use of IVIG found modest efficacy.[4]
3. Intervention for CRPS should follow a stepwise progression of more invasive procedures if the therapies are only partially or sub-optimally effective.[2]
   a. Minimally invasive: sympathetic nerve blocks, IV regional nerve blocks, somatic nerve blocks
   b. More invasive therapy: implantable drug infusion therapy, neurostimulation therapy
   c. Experimental therapy: sympathectomy, motor cortex stimulation
4. We recommend obtaining preoperative MR imaging of the thoracic or cervical spine, depending on the index levels, prior to implantation of a spinal cord stimulator device, as any critical stenosis might require decompression to facilitate safe placement of an electrode.
5. Careful review of the surgical and procedural history should be performed. Often extensive surgeries may add procedural difficulties or even preclude safe placement of the electrode. All relevant preoperative imaging should be carefully evaluated. Prior scarring and incisions may require adjustments in planning the entry of the electrode and placement of the impulse generator.

Oral Boards Review—Operative Management Pearls

1. If the patient is undergoing implantation under general anaesthesia, monitoring of motor and sensory potentials is critical. Midline placement of

the paddle can be assessed by monitoring EMG potentials, as well as somatosensory collision. Intermitted monitoring of motor and sensory potentials is recommended during adjustments of the epidural dorsal paddle.

2. During paddle placement difficulty in midline placement after several attempts should indicate a need for a skip laminotomy above the entry level.
3. Serial fluoroscopic imaging is recommended to ensure no movement of the electrode occurs during anchoring and tunneling of the electrode leads. We obtain postoperative X-rays as a baseline for comparison if problems develop later and hardware migration needs to be ruled out.

Pivot Points

1. Every patient should undergo neuropsychological evaluation prior to implantation of a SCS device. There is a high incidence of comorbid psychiatric conditions with CRPS. Furthermore, insurance companies will not approve coverage of SCS implantation without a preoperative neuropsychiatric evaluation.
2. Each patient should undergo a spinal cord stimulator trial with a greater than 50% relief in pain symptoms prior to permanent implantation of a device.
3. Paddle lead is preferred over percutaneous leads placement in patients with concomitant axial pain symptoms. In patients with coagulopathies and significant comorbidities, however percutaneous leads are preferred.

Aftercare and Follow-Up

At the end of the surgical procedure the patient was admitted overnight and discharged the following day. We typically obtain post-operative cervical X-rays to check placement and as a baseline for future reference. We then turn on the stimulator the day after surgery. Post-operatively she reported good coverage of her pain areas. Her immediate post-operative course was unremarkable, her sutures were removed, and her wounds healed well (Figure 21.1).

Complications and Management

Although she initially did well, after several months her efficacy was limited by the positionality of the device; that is, she needed to extend her neck to feel relief regardless of whether her stimulation was paresthesia or subparesthesia. It was then decided to revise her system to an epidural paddle system (Figure 21.2). Again the immediate post-operative period was unremarkable. She had no major issues in the immediate period afterward and had some improvement in her functional capabilities with further PT.

Oral Boards Review—Complications Pearls

1. Complications of placement of SCS are well known and include hardware migration, erosion, and infection. The overall complication rate ranges from

30 to 40% in reported literature, with a 0 to 10% infection rate and a 30 to 40% hardware complication rate.[5,6] Even rarer are neurologic complications, which are well below 1%.[7]

2. In a meta-analysis of 542 pts, surgical paddle versus percutaneous placement showed no significant difference in terms of hardware migration or hardware failure. Loss of efficacy was noted only among the percutaneous SCS placements. There was a statistically significant difference in regard to pain and wound complication rates between percutaneous and surgical paddle placement. Percutaneous was associated with fewer wound complications and less hardware site pain.[6]
3. More minimal techniques therefore appear to decrease wound complications. Techniques noted to reduce hardware complications include meticulous use of anchoring devices sutured to fascia and the use of strain relief loops to prevent migration.

Evidence and Outcomes

Treatment of CRPS is, for the most part, disappointing and not well studied. There are currently limited prospective studies on effective pharmacological treatment regimens or minimally invasive interventions for CRPS. More invasive interventions for CRPS with neuromodulation (i.e. spinal cord stimulation) have noted reasonable short-term effectiveness.[2] In a prospective randomized study, Kemler et al. studied 54 patients with CRPS type I who were randomized to receive spinal cord stimulation with physical therapy (SCS + PT, 31 pts) or physical therapy alone (PT, 18 pts). From 6 months to 3 years post-operative pain scores (VAS and global pain scores) were statistically significant between

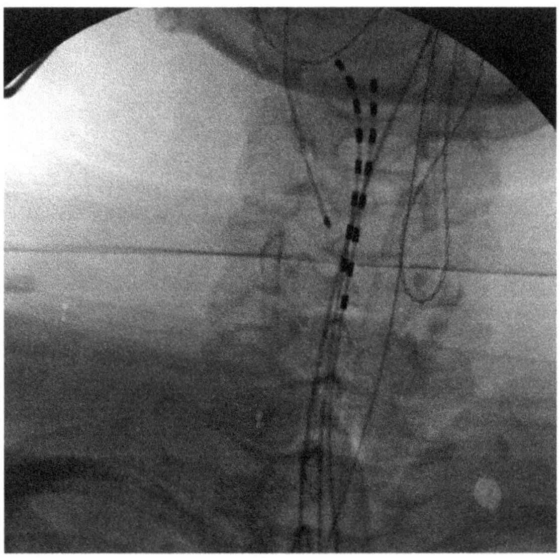

Figure 21.1. AP cervical X-ray showing placement of cervical percutaneous electrode. Left lead shows typical blooming flower configuration in order to capture the upper cervical roots for neck pain coverage. Here we mimicked the trial, which resulted in optimal coverage with the right lead in the midline.

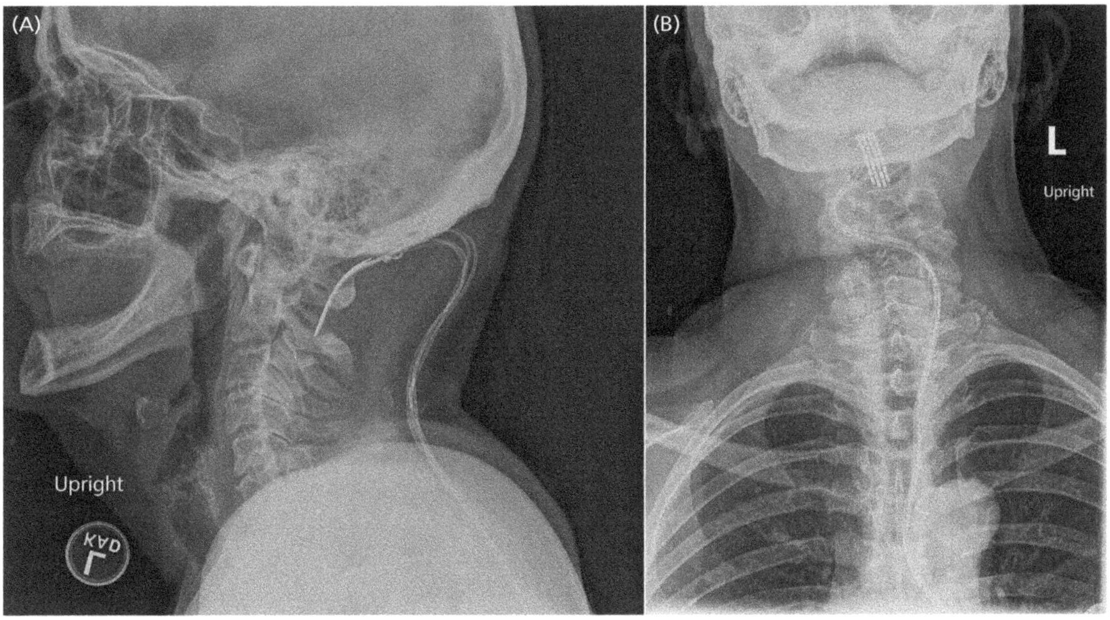

Figure 21.2. Cervical lateral and AP X-rays showing placement of cervical SCS paddle. Paddle placement is typically retrograde, since there is more space in the upper cervical spine.

the SCS + PT and PT groups in both intention to treat (ITT) and final analysis groups. After 3 years there was no statistically significant difference in the treatment groups in terms of pain scores and functional quality of life measures (Nottingham Health Profile, EQ-5D, and Sickness Impact Prolife-68). At 5 years post-operative follow-up reduction of VAS scores from SCS+PT compared to PT alone were −1.7 to −1.0, respectively, and were not statistically significant. This was postulated to occur from two likely independent reasons: first is that CRPS patients will improve with PT only; and second is that the efficacy of SCS may wane over time or patients may become noncompliant. The study showed a complications rate of approximately 40%. However, when asked at final follow-up, 19 of the 20 patients (95%) with SCS remaining stated that they would undergo the same treatment for the same result.[8] Furthermore, advances in SCS programing with high-frequency and burst-frequency stimulation (prior studies used tonic stimulation) are currently under investigation. These advanced programing methods can be used to salvage or extend the efficacy of SCS-treated patients who experienced lost treatment effect over time.

Recently, dorsal root ganglion (DRG) stimulation has shown promise to help patients with CRPS (Figure 21.3). Our understanding of the role of the DRG in chronic pain pathogenesis and its anatomical location has made it a recent neural target for the treatment of CRPS. The DRG is composed of sensory nerve cell bodies within the epidural space and is involved in transmitting pain to the central nervous system (CNS). In DRG stimulation, an electrical lead, connected by 4 electrode contacts, is placed on the DRG and a pulse generator is implanted into the lower back or into the abdominal wall. The mechanism of action can be explained by animal studies, which show that electrical stimulation of the DRG decreases the generation and propagation of action potentials. The authors concluded that the analgesic effect of DRG stimulation was due to reduced neuronal excitability, which blocked the transmission of pain to the CNS.[9]

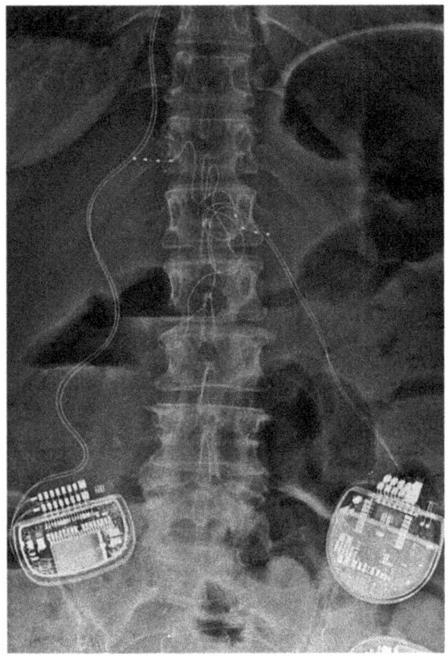

Figure 21.3. AP X-ray of lumbar spine, demonstrating an example of a DRG stimulator implant with DRG leads were ideally placed.

There has been a small, but encouraging, amount of research showing that DRG stimulation is safe and effective in treating chronic pain conditions.[10,11] One case series showed that 71.4% of CRPS patients who received DRG stimulation achieved at least 50% pain reduction after 6 months.[10] Most promising has been a prospective, multicenter, randomized control trial in 152 subjects in which patients received either SCS or DRG stimulation for the treatment of neuropathic lower-extremity pain due to CRPS or causalgia. Patients who received DRG stimulation showed a greater improvement in pain relief and treatment success at 3 months (81.2%) than those who had SCS (55.7%, $P < 0.001$). In addition, the patients who received DRG stimulation showed significantly greater improvements in mood disturbance, physical function, social function, and general health, as measured by various scales. However, this study did reveal a higher amount of non-serious procedure-related events in the DRG arm (46%) as compared with the SCS group (26%). The authors attributed this discrepancy to the fact that DRG stimulation required more leads and a longer average procedure time. With further experience in implantation of DRG stimulators and technical and procedural advances, there will inherently be fewer procedure-related complications.[12] Of note, DRG stimulation cannot be used in the cervical region. Overall, DRG stimulation has more precise targeting, provides higher pain relief, and shows greater improvements in overall patient health than SCS. Whether long-term efficacy will be maintained remains to be seen.

Conclusion

Management of CRPS should be multidisciplinary, with the ultimate goal of restoring function in the involved limb. Although studies are limited, neuromodulation via SCS remains of value in the management of CRPS, and advances in SCS programing with high-frequency and burst-frequency programs are currently under investigation. DRG stimulation may ultimately prove to be more efficacious as its technology and procedural technique advances; only time will tell.

Further Reading

1. Goh E, Chidambaram S, Ma D. Complex regional pain syndrome: a recent update. *Burns Trauma*. Jan 19 2017;5:2.
2. Harden RN, Oaklander AL, Burton AW, et al. Complex regional pain syndrome: practical diagnostic and treatment guidelines, 4th ed. *Pain Med*. Feb 2013(14):180–229.
3. Beydoun A. Neuropathic pain: from mechanisms to treatment strategies. *J Pain Symptom Manage*. 2003;25:S1–3.
4. Goebel A, Baranowski A, Maurer K. Intravenous immunoglobulin treatment of the complex regional pain syndrome: a randomized trial. *Ann Intern Med*. 2010(152):152–158.
5. Turner JA, Loeser JD, Bell KG. Spinal cord stimulation for chronic low back pain: a systematic literature synthesis. *Neurosurgery*. Dec 1995;37(6):1088–1096.
6. Shamji MF, Westwick HJ, Heary RF. Complications related to the use of spinal cord stimulation for managing persistent postoperative neuropathic pain after lumbar spinal surgery. *Neurosurg Focus*. Oct 2015;39(4):E15.
7. Levy R, Henderson J, Slavin K, et al. Incidence and avoidance of neurologic complications with paddle type spinal cord stimulation leads. *Neuromodulation*. Sept 2011;14(5):412–422.
8. Kemler MA, Vet HC, Barendse GA, Wildenberg FA, Kleef M. Effect of spinal cord stimulation for chronic complex regional pain syndrome Type I: five-year final follow-up of patients in a randomized controlled trial. *J Neurosurg*. Feb 2008;108(2):292–298.
9. Koopmeiners AS, Mueller S, Kramer J, Hogan QH. Effect of electrical field stimulation on dorsal root ganglion neuronal function. *Neuromodulation*. 2013;16:304–311.
10. Deer TR, Grigsby E, Weiner RL, Wilcosky B, Kramer JM. A prospective study of dorsal root ganglion stimulation for the relief of chronic pain. *Neuromodulation*. 2013;16:67–72.
11. VanBuyten JP, Smet I, Liem L, Russo M, Huygen F. Stimulation of dorsal root Ganglia for the management of complex regional pain syndrome: a prospective case series. *Pain Pract*. 2015;15:208–216.
12. Deer T, Levy R, Kramer J, et al. Dorsal root ganglion stimulation yielded higher treatment success rate for complex regional pain syndrome and causalgia at 3 and 12 months: a randomized comparative trial. *Pain*. Apr 2017;158(4):669.

Post-Stroke Intractable Pain

Innocent Njoku and Julie G. Pilitsis

22

Case Presentation

A 50-year-old male suffered from a right thalamic stroke with subsequent left-sided weakness and pain. After physical rehabilitation over the course of a 5-month period, his physical symptoms improved. However, his pain persisted despite maximum medication therapy including pregabalin, nitrazepam, nortiptyline, and dipyridamole. His neuropathic pain worsened over the following 7 years. On neurological exam, he experienced pain over his left face, neck, arm, and leg. He was noted to have corresponding allodynia.

Questions

1. What is the likely diagnosis?
2. What are appropriate diagnostic/screening tools used to discriminate possible etiologies of the diagnosis?
3. What are the most appropriate anatomical areas to image?

Assessment and Planning

The working diagnosis was central post-stroke pain (CPSP) syndrome and magnetic resonance imaging (MRI) if the brain revealed a right thalamic infarct. CPSP, previously known as thalamic pain syndrome, is a chronic, complex, disabling pain syndrome characterized by pain and temperature sensation abnormalities after a cerebrovascular infarct or hemorrhage. In this case, the diagnosis was clear; however, CPSP may be more difficult to diagnose, depending on presentation and region of the body affected. Other diagnoses may include spinal cord injury, post-herpetic neuralgia, and trigeminal neuropathic pain. When assessing patients for possible (sub)cortical neurosurgical treatment for CPSP, the following criteria should be met: (1) prior treatment had failed to provide relief; (2) no untreated psychological disorders; and (3) no contraindications to surgery. Pharmacological treatments, including NSAIDS, opioids, alpha 2 adrenergic agonists, antiepileptic drugs, muscle relaxant, and topical analgesics, can be used. Other treatment modalities include behavior modification treatments, psychotherapy, aerobic exercise, acupuncture, and physical and occupational therapy. Patient selection should involve a multidisciplinary team consisting of a pain specialist, neuropsychologist, and neurosurgeon. Comprehensive neuropsychologic evaluation is helpful to evaluate untreated depression and anxiety, borderline personality disorder, and dependence/addiction to pain medications.

Oral Boards Review—Diagnostic Pearls and Patient Selection

1. Physical findings in patients with CPSP may include hemiparesis/hemiplegia, hyperesthesia, or hypoesthesia on the contralateral side. Patients may also have impaired pinprick, temperature, and touch sensation on examination. Vibration and joint proprioception are less commonly affected.
2. A thorough psychological screening is also important for patient selection in neuromodulation.

Questions

1. How do clinical/radiological/screening tests affect surgical planning?
2. What are preoperative considerations to consider when deciding on a treatment plan?

Decision Making

CPSP is seen in the setting of known infarcts and hemorrhages and less commonly in patients who are unaware that they have had an event because it was purely sensory. An MRI of the brain will help confirm the diagnosis of thalamic and/or brainstem infarct. Theoretically, classification of pain can help determine the mode and targets for stimulation. Typically, the PAG matter is targeted for chronic nociceptive pain while the VP thalamus and motor cortex are targets for neuropathic pain. However, in reality, many patients have a component of both types of pain. In patients with hemibody pain, DBS is preferred to MCS as the homunculus related to the leg on the motor cortex is interhemispheric and thus unamenable to epidural MCS.

The target for PAG is x: 2–3 mm lateral to the third ventricle; y: 10 mm posterior to the mid-commissural point; and z: level of posterior commissure. Its pertinent anatomical boundaries in the midbrain include the medial lemniscus laterally, superior colliculus inferoposteriorly, and the red nucleus inferoanteriorly. Somatosensory thalamus stimulation targets are located in the contralateral somatosensory thalamus. Facial deafferentation pain is localized to the ventral posterior medial (VPM) nucleus while extremity deafferentation pain is localized in the ventral posterior lateral (VPL) nucleus. Targets are found 10–13 mm posterior to the mid-commissural point and from 5 mm below to 2 mm above it. The VPM thalamus is midway between the lateral wall of the third ventricle and the internal capsule; the arm area of VPL is 2–3 mm medial to the internal capsule, and the leg area of VPL 1–2 mm medial to the internal capsule. The sensory thalamus is bordered by centromedian-parafascicular complex medially; the internal capsule laterally; the thalamic fasciculus, zona incerta, and subthalamic nucleus inferiorly; the thalamic nucleus ventralis intermedius anteriorly; and the pulvinar thalamic nucleus posteriorly. PAG and VP remain the most common targets used for modulation of chronic pain.

When considering MCS, functional MRI has been used to help identify specific regions of the motor cortex underlying various functional territories. Increased blood oxygenation on fMRI, corresponding to increased neuronal activity, can by correlated with structural MRI for intraoperative planning and navigation. Often this is used in combination with neuronavigation and electrophysiological monitoring to localize the motor cortex. See chapter 19, "Trigeminal Neuropathic Pain," for further details.

Questions

1. What are the technical caveats of subcortical versus cortical electrical stimulation?
2. Why is a trial period necessary prior to permanent placement?

Surgical Procedure

The three fundamental aspects of DBS include defining the target, placement of electrodes, and physiological testing following placement. DBS leads are placed with the patient under local sedation. Briefly, a stereotactic frame is attached to the patient's head and one or two burr holes are made depending on whether a unilateral or a bilateral procedure is performed. Typically, leads are placed into both the PAG and the VPL/VPM through a single burr hole (Figure 22.1). Microelectrode recording (MER) may be used to differentiate between gray and white matter and microstimulation may be used to induce side effects prior to placing the leads. Feelings of relaxation and warmth have been noted with stimulation of PAG/PVG matter and paresthesias with VP stimulation. Once the lead location is confirmed, the incision is closed and a 5–7 day trial of stimulation obtained by connecting the leads to external cables. Stimulation parameters differ among authors, but PAG stimulation in a recent case series was found to be most effective at a voltage of 1–5 V, a pulse width of 30–90 microseconds, and a frequency of 5–15 Hz; VPL/VPM stimulation parameters were found to be ideal at a voltage of 3–8 V, pulse width of 0.1–1 msec, and 20–100 Hz. Devices are permanently implanted in patients who demonstrated > 50% pain relief.

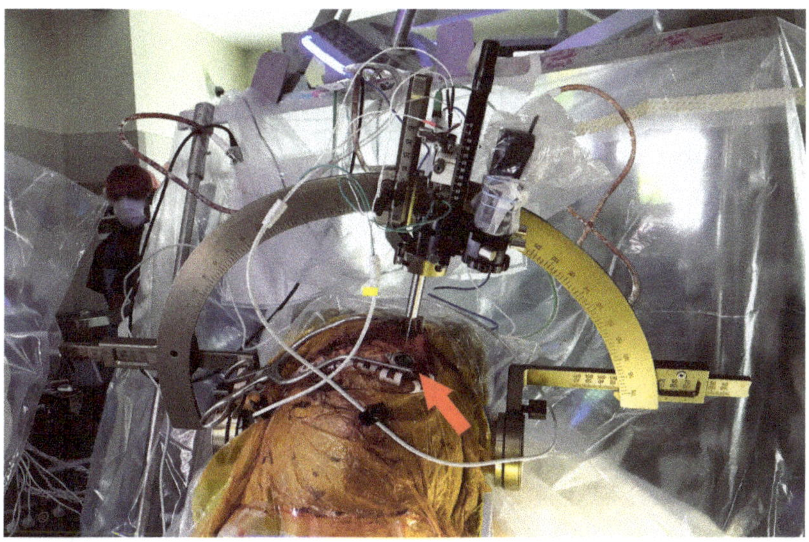

Figure 22.1. Intraoperative image of DBS with demonstration of burrhole (arrow) and stereotactic frame.

MCS is performed through a craniotomy using somatosensory evoked potential mapping and intraoperative navigation with fMRI. Typically, the electrodes are placed epidurally. There have been some reports of subdural placement as lower stimulation intensity is needed; however, seizure incidence is anecdotally higher. See chapter 19 for more details.

Oral Boards Review—Management Pearls

1. Deep brain stimulation should be considered only after patients have failed multimodality medical management.
2. Most patients will receive both PAG and VP leads, as it is often difficult to clinically discern between nociceptive and neuropathic pain in these patients.

Pivot Point

1. If a patient presents with sudden focal neurological changes immediately postoperatively, urgent diagnostic imaging is indicated to rule out hemorrhage. In general, DBS intracranial hemorrhages are able to be managed non-operatively except in rare cases of large or extra-axial hematomas.
2. If infection is suspected, appropriate antibiotics should be initiated immediately. Partial or complete lead/hardware removal may be indicated.
3. If the patient reports sudden loss of efficacy, device/hardware malfunction should be considered. Mechanical stress may result in lead fracture, extension cable, or generator failure. The device should be interrogated to check impedances.

Aftercare

A postoperative neurological exam is crucial to monitor neurological function. Immediate postoperative images should be obtained in the advent of focal neurological deficits. In addition, perioperative prophylactic antibiotics should be routinely administered to avoid complications relating to infection. Superficial infections may be managed, in selected cases, in a non-operative and conservative fashion with close monitoring and a short course (1–2 weeks) of antibiotics. In the event of a deep infection involving the hardware or the brain tissue, many authors elect to remove all hardware. A CT head with neuronavigation protocol should be obtained, prior to removing the device in case of infection, when planning for reimplantation.

In cases where patients report loss of efficacy, the device itself should be investigated. A high impedance may be consistent with a lead fracture or a suboptimal connection. X-rays of the entire system may provide further guidance concerning lead fracture and/or migration.

Complications and Management

Both DBS and MCS are invasive surgical procedures with potential complications that can be significant. The most serious reported event is intracranial hemorrhage. In most cases, these hemorrhages are small and appropriate for medical management. In cases of large hemorrhage, surgery may be indicated. Other complications include infection, migraines, erosion of hardware, psychosis, lead migration/misplacement, and post-operative seizures. Infections are the most common complication with DBS. Seizures are the most frequent complication with MCS. In this regard, patients are typically maintained on anticonvulsant medication while voltage parameters are explored. Other, less common complications documented in MCS include pain due to stimulation of the dura and dysesthesias.

Oral Boards Review—Complications Pearls

1. Careful peri-operative and long-term follow-up will limit complications with intracranial neuromodulation procedures.
2. Post-operative seizures may occur during programming of MCS and necessitate temporary anti-epileptic management.
3. If a patient experiences unwanted stimulation effects, including persistent paresthesias, muscle pulling, and /or behavioral changes, the device should be shut off. If the symptoms resolve with DBS turned off, reprogramming should be attempted.

Evidence and Outcomes

VPL/VPM and PAG DBS have demonstrated significant pain relief in several studies and are indicated in patients with refractory pain. Patients with nociceptive pain responded favorably to bilateral PAG/PVG stimulation. In one study, Hosobuchi et al. showed that 77% of patients experience long-term (2 years) pain relief in a cohort of 65 patients with chronic pain syndrome and bilateral implantation of electrodes in the PAG/PVG matter. In initial studies targeting the VPL/VPM, 60–70% of patients expressed long-term (> 1 year) pain relief following isolated VP DBS placement. In a smaller subgroup of patients with neuropathic pain, simultaneous VPM/VPL and PAG stimulation achieved long-term pain relief.

MCS has been employed most commonly to treat trigeminal neuropathic pain with good efficacy as compared to other central pain syndromes. The face is represented by a large territory on the motor cortex and is easily stimulated by electrode contact. Historically, studies have demonstrated 60–80% response rates in long-term pain relief in patients with trigeminal neuropathic pain. DBS is considered more appropriate for certain pain etiologies—specifically those with hemi-body refractory pain.

Further Reading

Hadded, AR, Ughratdar K, Ashkan A. A single thalamic target for deep brain stimulation to treat hemi-body pain syndrome. Acta Neurochirurgica. 2015; 157(9):1519–1523.

Hosobuchi Y. Subcortical electrical stimulation for control of intractable pain humans. Report of 122 cases. J Neurosurg. 1986;164(4):543–553.

Kumar K, Toth C, Nath RK. Deep brain stimulation for intractable pain: a 15-year experience. Neurosurgery. 1997 April; 40 (4):736–746.

Morishita T, FOote KD, Burdock AP, Katayama Y, Yamamoto T, Frucht SJ, Okun MS. Identification and management of deep brain stimulation intra- and postoperative urgencies emergencies. Parkinsonism Relat Disord. 2010; 16 (3):153–162.

Nguyen JP, Lefaucher JP, Le Guerinel C, Eizenbaum JF, Nakano N, Carpentier A, Brugieres P, Pollin B, Rostaing S, Keravel Y. Motor cortex stimulation in the treatment of central and neuropathic pain. Archives of Medical Research. 2000; 31 (3):263–265.

Parma VK, Gee L, Smith H, Pilitsis JG. Supraspinal stimulation for treatment of refractory pain. Clinical Neurology and Neurosurgery. 2013; 123:155–163.

Index

Note: Tables and figures are indicated *t*, and *f*, following the page/paragraph number

For the benefit of digital users, indexed terms that span two pages (e.g., 52–53) may, on occasion, appear on only one of those pages.

www.ingramcontent.com/pod-product-compliance
Lightning Source LLC
Chambersburg PA
CBHW052128160126
38387CB00036B/1327
* 9 7 8 0 1 9 0 8 8 7 6 7 4 *